THE
IVF REVOLUTION

Other books from Vermilion
by Professor Robert Winston

INFERTILITY

THE
IVF
REVOLUTION

*The Definitive Guide to Assisted
Reproductive Techniques*

Professor Robert Winston

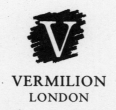

VERMILION
LONDON

This book is dedicated to four colleagues who,
in their different ways, have done so much in their attempts
to alleviate the pain of those suffering with fertility problems:

Karin Dawson
Jennie Hunt
Raul Margara
Geoffrey Trew

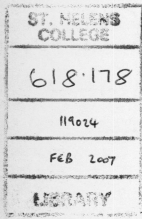
1 3 5 7 9 10 8 6 4 2

First published in the United Kingdom in 1999 by Vermilion
an imprint of Ebury Press
Random House
20 Vauxhall Bridge Road
London SW1V 2SA

Random House Australia (Pty) Limited
20 Alfred Street, Milsons Point, Sydney,
New South Wales 2061, Australia

Random House New Zealand Limited
18 Poland Road, Glenfield,
Auckland 10, New Zealand

Random House South Africa (Pty) Limited
Endulini, 5A Jubilee Road,
Parktown 2193, South Africa

Random House UK Limited Reg. No. 954009

A CIP catalogue for this book is available from the British Library

ISBN: 0 09 181682 3

Printed and bound in Great Britain by Mackays of Chatham plc, Kent

Contents

Preface

This book deals with that field of medicine loosely called 'assisted reproduction'. Essentially, there are three aspects to it. First, it involves methods of treatment to achieve pregnancy – *in vitro* fertilisation, insemination with sperm and treatment with donated eggs of embryos – which avoid the need for sex. This is hardly natural and this is why these treatments are so often considered controversial, especially by many religious people. Secondly, each of these treatments gives doctors and scientists access to the very beginnings of life – either the embryo itself, or the egg and sperm. To many people, this represents the risk of humans manipulating God-given or natural processes. Thirdly, all assisted reproductive treatments are episodic. Each is a 'one-shot' treatment. If the treatment works, pregnancy is immediate; if it fails, the person treated is not only not pregnant, but physically unchanged, and the medical condition which gave rise to the reproductive problem is unaltered. Consequently, these treatments raise great expectations and can produce immediate happiness, but can also cause great stress and distress.

The IVF Revolution is an attempt to look at some of these issues and to assess how IVF might be improved. One major concern is that, in too many instances, people are being put through these complex treatments without any clear idea of why they are needed. Too often, no serious attempt to make a proper diagnosis has been made. This is doubly damaging: first, if the treatment doesn't work, the infertile person is no better off and secondly, they may be made even more unhappy because the reason for failure is not understood. It surely must be every person's right to have a reasonable idea of what is wrong before treatment is contemplated.

So, at one level, medical management of reproductive disorders is still quite crude but, at the same time, technology is becoming increasingly sophisticated. We are starting to diagnose and prevent the development of certain hereditary diseases such as muscular distrophy and cystic fibrosis, before the embryo has even implanted. We can already choose the sex of a child by selecting fertilised eggs or by influencing fertilisation. Soon, we may be able to clone a human. It may eventually be possible to alter the genetic characteristics of our children and 'enhance' attributes – such as intelligence, strength, beauty – that we see as desirable.

There are other reasons why so many people are critical of modern reproductive technology. Many criticise infertility treatment because they see it as a waste of resources. Some point to the fact that the world already contains 5.9 billion people. If the current rate of childbirth on this planet is maintained, there will be over 250 billion people within the next 100 years. How can infertility treatments be justified when the world's resources are apparently so severely threatened? As we shall see in this book, infertility treatment, the new reproductive technologies and better health care generally may paradoxically offer the salvation of this planet.

Chief among the core human impulses is the desire to have children. Nothing will alter the fact that the most important thing that most people do in their lives is to bring a child into the world. It changes our lives completely, and it reaffirms the cycle of life and our place in it. Having children makes us feel a part of the world yet many people are denied this vital experience. The blow of discovering that one is infertile is heavy. It is unequalled in any sphere of life because for those who suffer it, it often feels as if, for no good reason, they have been judged inadequate by some supreme will of the heavens. Those who are infertile are not only unable to feel and express the emotions that parenthood brings, they are also barred from contributing to the continuity of human existence. Having a child brings parents a kind of immortality which childless couples may only watch with envy.

Cures for infertility and recipes for preventing the birth of children with defects are as old as the Bible. But in the last few decades it has been possible to offer evidence-based treatments for infertile couples. There is never a guarantee of success and the treatments, especially those involving assisted reproduction, tend to be complex and puzzling. It is sometimes difficult to understand how they are actually done; why they succeed or fail is often even more enigmatic.

The IVF Revolution is written for those people who are experiencing problems in having a child. I hope that it will give them a better under-standing of what is wrong, and how they can help improve their treatment. It is also written as a manual of IVF for a much wider audience. Apart from healthcare professionals, there are many people who are concerned with our increasing ability to manipulated reproduc-tion. The fact that humans potentially can change the basis of life seems, quite reasonably, a serious threat to family values – not to say human values. These issues are too often handled in the hope of deliberately causing alarm or controversy.

The science of reproduction should be a force for good in this century to come. Not only will it greatly improve family life for many millions, it could contribute hugely to the health and welfare of our future children. In addition, the study of human embryology has huge implications for the improvement of medicine. If properly used during the next 100 years, this science could contribute to finding better treatments for many adult diseases. *In vitro* fertilisation is indeed a revolution. It is up to us, by improving our understanding of all that it involves, to ensure that this revolution is controlled and that it leads to the improvement of the human condition.

Professor Robert Winston
March 1999

1
In vitro fertilisation

What is IVF?

IVF is the process by which egg and sperm are mixed in a small plastic or glass container outside the body and then placed in a woman's uterus after fertilisation. It usually involves the removal of eggs from the woman's ovary and the collection of sperm from her partner. The embryo, which results from fertilisation in the laboratory, is transferred to the woman's uterus about two to five days later. At this stage, long before any organs have formed, it is still invisible to the naked eye and consists of only a few cells.

In vitro fertilisation (IVF) has had huge publicity and has gained a false reputation as the panacea for infertility. In practice it is one of the most demanding of all the procedures in reproductive medicine and is less successful than some alternatives. Strictly speaking, IVF is not even a 'treatment' for infertility as it does not alter the underlying cause of infertility. It is simply a one-off attempt to help someone who is infertile to have a baby. The attempt can be repeated several times, but the basic cause of infertility remains.

Because IVF does not change the underlying causes of infertility, it is best where possible to seek therapy which may improve the chances of becoming pregnant naturally. But there is no doubt that IVF has revolutionised the treatment of infertile people and increased our knowledge about many aspects of what causes infertility.

There are several often-used medical phrases with which it is well to be familiar:

In vitro fertilisation means literally 'fertilisation in glassware' (from the Latin *vitrum*), although glassware is hardly ever used now in IVF clinics. Because of the need for absolute cleanliness and the impossibility of washing glass thoroughly enough, doctors have mostly used disposable plastic containers and equipment, which are used once and then thrown away.

Embryo transfer describes the process by which the embryo is put into the mother's uterus.

Extra-corporeal fertilisation means fertilisation outside the body – it is merely a superfluous term for those too stubborn to say IVF.

IVF is often confused with artificial insemination (AI) which is completely different. Artificial insemination refers to conception that does not take place by sexual intercourse. It involves a doctor or nurse placing sperm directly into a woman's vagina or uterus with a syringe or using some other artificial method; fertilisation then occurs in the woman's fallopian tube in the normal way.

It is important to realise that IVF is not always the ideal treatment for most infertility patients. Certainly it should not be the first option to be considered. More than half the women referred to IVF clinics could be better treated by alternatives. Too frequently no systematic assessment of the medical condition of the patient is made at the outset. There is a real need for referring General Practitioners (GPs) to make better judgements as to whether a patient would most benefit from IVF treatment, rather than an alternative. Often patients themselves push for IVF when there may be a more suitable, possibly cheaper, treatment.

Sadly, even specialists in reproductive medicine are tending to refer patients for IVF before it is proved to be necessary. Far too many couples enter an *in vitro* fertilisation programme before complete medical investigation. This is doubly unfortunate. It means that the IVF itself is more likely to fail because there may be an underlying condition – for example, a uterine abnormality – which needs treatment and may prevent a pregnancy implanting with or without IVF. It also means that treatment of the actual cause is avoided, when this might give a much better chance than IVF of a pregnancy. I cannot overstate the importance of diagnosing the true cause of infertility. The investigations which should be done before IVF are discussed at length in the next chapter.

When is IVF appropriate?

In general IVF should be considered only once a diagnosis is reached. It is an appropriate treatment in the following situations:

- When the fallopian tubes are so badly damaged that tubal surgery has failed or where tubal damage is so bad that surgery is not worth contemplating. Under these circumstances IVF really is the only satisfactory treatment, because it bypasses the fallopian tubes. Unfortunately, IVF is too often used when there is relatively minor damage of the fallopian tubes. Where this is the case it is well worth the patient asking her GP to seek an expert opinion as to whether tubal surgery might be more justified from one with a great deal of experience in managing tubal disease.

- A man has an abnormal or low sperm count but the sperm are still potentially capable of fertilising an egg. IVF is undoubtedly the ideal course of action in such circumstances. Manipulation of the sperm in the laboratory may make the sperm much more likely to fertilise an egg. Alternatively one of the modern, assisted reproductive techniques such as sperm microinjection may be useful. Using this technique, a single sperm is picked up under the microscope and then injected directly into the egg (see page 66).

- For many women who are not ovulating and where attempts to use drugs to stimulate ovulation have failed IVF is useful. Probably the most significant cause of this is polycystic ovary disease. However, there are other situations where the ovaries are capable of producing an egg but do not do so regularly. IVF is much less valuable for women who are not ovulating and who are incapable of producing an egg, or for those who produce eggs of very poor quality, usually only after very heavy stimulation (see page 5). Under these circumstances taking a donor egg from another woman may be the only realistic alternative.

- For a number of women with endometriosis (where the lining of the uterus, the endometrium, grows not only in the uterus but also in the abdomen leading to adhesions or severe scarring of the tubes) IVF is a highly successful treatment. However, it must be remembered that the stimulation required to persuade the ovaries to give up a number of eggs does increase a woman's own natural circulating hormone level of oestrogen, which in turn can stimulate the endometriosis and make it more severe. This generally is not a problem, but it is not uncommon for women with endometriosis to find that symptoms of pain and irregular bleeding increase after an unsuccessful IVF treatment. Endometriosis may be treated surgically and by other means. In certain circumstances, this is more likely to be a successful treatment for infertility than IVF.

- In cases of unexplained infertility, where proper attempts to diagnose infertility have been unsuccessful and the condition remains un-explained, IVF is highly valuable. In general, IVF has a good success rate in cases of unexplained infertility. However, in older women, where the unexplained infertility may actually be due to the ovaries being incapable of producing normal eggs, IVF is much less likely to be successful.

- When there is a problem with the sub-cervix or severe scarring of the top of the vagina (usually after surgery), IVF may be quite helpful. Because IVF bypasses the cervical canal, by introducing embryos directly into the uterine cavity it is frequently a successful treatment for these conditions.
- When there are multiple factors causing infertility, usually affecting both the man and the woman there is no doubt that IVF is by far the most effective treatment. If there is a minor sperm problem for example combined with a minor problem in the fallopian tubes, then IVF greatly increases the chances of fertilisation and pregnancy. There are many other examples of combined infertility of this kind which are greatly helped by using IVF treatment.
- For those couples who are at relatively high risk of having genetically abnormal babies IVF is now used frequently. Using preimplantation genetic diagnosis (page 83), an assessment of whether or not a particular embryo is free of a genetic defect can be made. With this advanced technology, a healthy embryo can then be put in the mother's uterus where it may develop.

When is IVF inappropriate?

Unfortunately there are numerous couples for whom IVF fertilisation is likely to be of very little, if any, help at all:

- There is no treatment currently for a man who is producing no sperm at all. While it is true that even when there are no sperm in the seminal fluid, there may be sperm in the testes itself, this situation is relatively uncommon. If the testes are not producing any sperm, there is no chance at present of IVF working. The alternative is to consider using donor semen from a suitable donor: artificial insemination by donor (AID) or donor insemination (DI) (see page 44).
- When the uterus has been removed by hysterectomy, there is no prospect of bearing a child. For these women, the only possibility is adoption or, in exceptional circumstances, surrogacy. In very rare cases, it may be possible to take an egg from the ovaries (if these are still intact), fertilise it outside the body by IVF, and then produce a surrogate pregnancy in another woman. This approach, however, involves entering a legal and moral minefield. If the patient has very

severe scarring, or a serious abnormality of the uterus, particularly after surgery (for example for extensive or very large fibroids) pregnancy may be impossible.

- Some rare infections of the uterus such as tuberculosis make implantation and subsequent pregnancy impossible.
- Where severe adhesions inside the uterine cavity are largely obliterating it. This condition is called Asherman's syndrome. In its most severe, untreatable form, embryo transfer will fail and therefore IVF is generally not worth trying.
- When the ovaries are very scarred, extensively cystic or not capable of producing an egg because of scar tissue.
- When the ovaries are failing to produce any eggs at all or when women are in the older age group and post-menopausal. Under these circumstances the only possibility is receiving an egg from a donor.
- In some women there are severe bowel adhesions around the ovaries, making any form of egg collection a life-threatening procedure.

The IVF procedure

1 Testing a couple's suitability for treatment

Before treatment, and following routine fertility investigations, several specific tests should be carried out. Hormone levels should be carefully rechecked and measurements of the hormone Follicle Stimulating Hormone (FSH) taken. If the FSH is much above 10 units, then attempts to stimulate the ovaries may be a complete failure (see below). Sperm counts should be rechecked further to the preliminary diagnostic tests. Sperm function tests should be run and the motility of the sperm assessed. The uterine cavity should be examined if this has not been done recently. A probe such as a fine plastic tube should be passed through the cervix to make sure that an embryo transfer can be done without difficulty during the actual IVF treatment. In some units, the woman may also be given stimulatory drugs such as clomiphene as a test to make sure that her ovaries can respond to the drugs used during the IVF treatment cycle. This also enables the medical team to tailor the stimulation to an individual's needs.

2 Stimulation of the ovaries

A successful pregnancy is more likely to occur when more than one embryo is placed in the uterus at the same time. This is because so many human embryos, normally fertilised, miscarry at an early stage or do not develop into babies. To overcome this natural loss, several embryos are usually placed in the uterus simultaneously, if available. Under British law a maximum of three embryos can be transferred at the same time. There are no absolute restrictions in most other countries, including the USA. The increased risk of multiple pregnancy in these circumstances is not great, but is still high enough to be of serious concern. For this reason, more and more British units are now transferring only two embryos simultaneously.

On average, only about 60 per cent of eggs will be capable of being fertilised. Normally, therefore, several eggs are required to make sufficient embryos for transfer. In order to stimulate the ovaries to release more than the one egg, injections containing the hormone FSH are given. In exceptional cases up to forty eggs can be obtained with these drugs in one cycle but it is very rare for all of them to fertilise and turn into normal embryos. More frequently, the number of eggs produced is around ten to fifteen.

There are various ways in which the stimulatory dose of FSH may be given. Most frequently, the ovaries are first prepared by making them inactive. This requires giving a drug to induce a brief, temporary menopause for two or three weeks only. The drugs which make the ovary inactive work on the pituitary gland in the brain and usually prevent it from making its own natural FSH to stimulate the ovaries. Consequently the ovaries not only stop ovulating, but also stop producing follicles, the small round structures in which the eggs develop. This may seem a surprising approach, but in most women it then makes the ovary more sensitive to injections of FSH.

The process of ovarian suppression is most frequently started the day after the menstrual period starts. Generally speaking suppression is most reliably obtained when it is started immediately after a bleeding has commenced. However, in some units, very good results are obtained by starting in the second half of the menstrual cycle, usually one week before the period is due.

In Britain the drug most commonly used to suppress ovarian function is called Suprefact (Buserelin). This is normally sniffed every four to six hours throughout the day, usually one sniff into each nostril. Sniffing allows the drug to be very rapidly absorbed. Women who cannot sniff – perhaps because of a cold – or who get very poor absorption of the drug by sniffing it – can be given an injection, generally several times a day.

There are alternatives to drugs like Suprefact. A very similar effect can be gained by a single depot injection of a long-acting drug to suppress the ovaries. This approach is more popular in the United States and parts of Europe than it is in Britain, where short-acting drugs which require more injections are preferred, because they are usually more reliable and their effect much easier to reverse. (This is known as the 'long protocol'.)

Curiously, although all these drugs work by suppressing the pituitary function, in the first few days after their administration they very frequently stimulate it, so that the pituitary temporarily produces more FSH than is normal. This effect is utilised by some clinics and the external injections of FSH are given before the pituitary is suppressed so as to cut down the amount of FSH needed during the cycle. This particular approach, the so-called 'short protocol', may be particularly useful for women who do not respond well to injections of FSH (older women, for example).

A number of women do not respond very well to drugs which suppress the pituitary after first stimulating it. In consequence, the drug companies have been researching preparations which do not have to stimulate the pituitary in order to have a subsequent suppressing effect. At the time of writing, these drugs are being used experimentally and have just begun to appear on the market. At present there is no conclusive evidence to show whether they are better or worse than the drugs now most commonly prescribed.

Drugs to suppress the pituitary can cause side-effects. Some women feel quite tired, others have headaches, and some can get quite severe hot flushes. On rare occasions breakthrough bleeding can occur for a few days. While all these symptoms are certainly unpleasant, none is dangerous, and the main concern is that they make patients uncomfortable. The symptoms rapidly disappear when the drugs are stopped. On very rare occasions, the suppression of the pituitary function continues for a few weeks after stopping the drugs, and consequently some women have an irregular cycle or two after IVF.

Usually, within two weeks, the ovaries become completely suppressed. It is usual practice to confirm that the ovaries are totally suppressed by doing an ultrasound examination to show that no follicles are developing. A blood test may also be taken to make certain that very little oestrogen is being produced by the ovaries. This is evidence that the ovaries are satisfactorily quiescent.

Once the ovaries have been completely suppressed (usually after two weeks of administration using the 'long protocol') injections of FSH are given. Most widely used now are the recombinant FSH drugs Gonal F or

Puregon. These are given once daily by injection. (These drugs have virtually totally replaced the older drugs Pergonal and Metrodin. These were produced by extraction from the urine of menopausal women and frequently contained unwanted proteins, which occasionally cause adverse reactions.) The modern genetically engineered (recombinant) drugs appear to be a good deal safer but are probably no more effective. Sadly they are expensive. Older women, who generally never respond as well to ovarian stimulation as younger women, need more of these drugs. Consequently their treatment tends to be more expensive. The potential short-term and long-term risks involved with ovulatory drugs are discussed on page 159.

3 Assessing the development of the follicles and eggs

Egg collection is usually timed to coincide within a few hours of when the woman would normally be expected to ovulate. If eggs are not collected close to this time, they many not fertilise properly. Before ovulation, the follicles containing the egg gradually become responsive to luteinising hormone (LH). This is usually produced by the pituitary gland, but in women whose pituitary has been suppressed (with for example Buserelin) no LH is produced. Consequently a drug has to be given to mature the eggs sufficiently so that they are capable of being fertilised. This is given in the form of human chorionic gonadotrophin (HCG) approximately 36 hours before the egg collection is scheduled. HCG is given rather than LH itself, because it is as effective, and easier and cheaper to manufacture. Timing the injection of HCG is very important. If it is given too early, the egg may not mature properly; if it is given too late, the egg may be lost completely. This is why many clinics perform regular hormone tests, measuring oestrogen during stimulation. The level of oestrogen gives some indication of how well the follicles are responding to the FSH injections and therefore helps the timing of the HCG injections.

Ultrasound is also used to assess the response to stimulation. A high frequency sound source is used and the echoes are detected on a computer screen. It is generally done over several days and can be used to assess the swelling of the follicles. Nearly all clinics use vaginal ultrasound, which involves inserting a probe gently into the vagina. Most patients prefer this to abdominal ultrasound which requres the patient to drink large amounts of water. Women can also take an interest in what the doctor is seeing on the ultrasound monitor without having the discomfort of a full bladder. When the biggest follicle is about seventeen to twenty millimetres across, ovulation is imminent, and it is time to consider the HCG injection. In practice this is usually ten to fourteen days after starting FSH.

On very rare occasions clinics use so-called 'natural cycle' IVF. They will give no other stimulus to the ovaries beyond a single injection of HCG to trigger ovulation. Without stimulation usually only one egg can be collected. Natural cycle IVF is cheaper because FSH injections are expensive, and the transfer of one embryo avoids the risk of twins. However, as the number of transferred embryos is reduced the treatment is very much less successful. Natural cycle IVF usually has a success rate of less than three per cent.

4 Egg collection

On very rare occasions eggs are collected by laparoscopy. This requires a telescope to be inserted into the abdomen and a general anaesthetic is needed. However, in nearly all cases nowadays, eggs are collected with the aid of a vaginal ultrasound. The ultrasound probe gives a picture of each of the ovaries. A needle is then placed through the top of the vagina and guided into the ovary. Eggs are sucked from the follicles into a small test tube, and then handed to the embryologist to examine. This convenient technique frequently involves only a light general anaesthetic or a local anaesthetic with sedation. There is seldom any real pain.

However careful the doctor may be, it is not always possible to get all the eggs – or sometimes even a single egg – which have matured. But in good clinics 97 per cent of attempts at egg collection yield at least one egg, unless there is very severe disease of the ovaries. It is quite common to give an antibiotic for a few days after egg collection. This prevents infection then and during embryo transfer and will not harm any developing pregnancy.

Recovery after egg collection is usually very swift. Most women are able to leave the clinic within two to four hours of collection. There is usually very little pain or soreness, but because the anaesthetic may make some people light-headed, it is best to be accompanied from the clinic.

5 Egg culture, sperm preparation and fertilisation

Once the eggs have been collected, they are vulnerable to damage. They are carefully examined in special fluid used for handling eggs, under a microscope in the operating theatre where they have just been obtained. Once they have been assessed, they are immediately placed in another specially prepared fluid, known as the culture medium. The culture medium contains precisely measured amounts of the chemicals needed for the eggs to survive. It may also contain some of the woman's own serum previously obtained from a sample of her blood.

Culture media vary from unit to unit. However, all media have generally the same basic constituents – that is, the proteins, salts and sugars required for maintenance of fertilisation and early growth. Maternal serum may be added, because this provides a balance of the essential ingredients for life. By using the mother's own blood any infection from external sources can be ruled out. In the past many medical units, including my own, made up their own media. It is now widely accepted that media of sufficient purity can be bought from commercial sources.

The medium, with the eggs inside, is then put into an incubator which will keep the eggs at precisely the right temperature. The closely controlled conditions there should resemble as much as possible those of the body.

Meanwhile, shortly before the eggs are to be collected, the male partner will have been asked to produce semen by masturbation. A bedroom is available in most clinics for this purpose. Men often find this part of IVF disturbing, and the emotional pressure can often cause a man to fail to ejaculate. If this is likely to be a difficulty, it is possible to arrange to freeze and store semen samples well before treatment. But, unfortunately, frozen semen which has then been thawed out is not always likely to be as fertile as fresh semen.

Once the semen has been produced, the sperm are washed in special media and all débris commonly present in semen is removed. The total number of sperm are diluted in the laboratory, and their number counted under a microscope. Some time after egg collection, usually four to eight hours later, they will be mixed with the culture medium containing the eggs, which will then be returned to the incubator. Often there are last-minute problems with the sperm. They may be too few in number or too weak. Most IVF programmes need several thousand normal sperm to guarantee fertilisation of just one egg. If there are very few sperm, or if most of the sperm are not normal, then help to achieve fertilisation may be needed. In centres where the special equipment and training are available, this normally involves the microinjection of sperm into the egg (ICSI; see page 66).

6 Assessment of fertilisation

A good IVF unit will inspect the cultured eggs under a microscope about eighteen hours after they have been mixed with the sperm. This may be the only time at which it is possible to observe definite signs of fertilisation.

What the embryologist will be looking for are two pronuclei – the nucleus of the egg and the head of the fertilising sperm which can be seen in the centre of the egg – but only at this stage. Later than this and some eggs may divide into several cells without ever having been actually fertilised. This is known as 'parthenogenetic cleavage', and unless the cultured eggs have been carefully observed there is a risk that unfertilised, parthenogenetically cleaved eggs – which of course will not result in a pregnancy – may be transferred to the uterus. Sometimes, too, there may be abnormal fertilisation when more than one sperm penetrates the egg – leading to the development of three or even more eggs. This kind of 'polyspermic' fertilisation is more common when the eggs are abnormal in some way – or in the eggs of women in the older age group.

7 Embryo assessment

The embryos have usually divided into about two to four cells after 48 hours. At some time from now they will normally be ready to transfer to the uterus. An embryologist will check to make sure that they appear normal. If there are doubts about their development a further assessment may be made in 24 hours' time. In good units this extra wait does not affect the chances of a successful pregnancy. If an embryo seems seriously abnormal, it is discarded rather than risk a damaged pregnancy. In some clinics embryos are now being kept for longer than two or even three days outside the body. Occasionally they may be kept for up to five days by which time they have developed to the blastocyst stage. The reason for this is that the blastocyst, being further advanced in development, may be more likely to implant (see page 134).

All clinics assess embryo quality by looking at embryos down a microscope. This is an extremely imperfect way of predicting whether an embryo is capable of further development or not. A normal embryo tends to have divided into an equal number of cells which are of equal size and round and smooth. This is no guarantee of normality, but in general embryos which are cleaved equally are more likely to result in successful pregnancy. Some embryos may have an unequal number of cells and very often these cells are of unequal size. In general this is either because the embryo is dividing at the time of inspection or because the cells are fragmenting. If the latter is the case, then the embryo is less likely to produce a pregnancy. Some embryos are very fragmented, with many little pieces of unequal size and shape. In general, the more fragments, the less likely the embryo is to develop. However, even very abnormal-looking embryos are capable occasionally of producing a pregnancy and, surprisingly, an abnormal-looking embryo, if transferred to the womb, does not give an increased risk of an abnormal baby.

Far too many clinics, including our own, tend to reassure patients that their embryos are normal-looking. This is a mistake because even most normal-looking embryos are not capable of becoming a baby. It is rather like looking at somebody's face and saying that they look intelligent or stupid. In general, you cannot tell the quality of an embryo by looking at it down a microscope.

It is also true that embryos which are dividing faster than average are probably slightly more likely to be capable of becoming a baby. For example, if an embryo has divided into only two or three cells three days after fertilisation, then a pregnancy is less likely than if an embryo has divided into eight or ten cells. However, this is only a rule of thumb and even embryos which seem quite retarded in their development are capable of becoming completely normal healthy babies.

Only about one in five human embryos are capable of becoming a pregnancy. The reason for this is not clear. As so many human embryos stop developing the first three days after fertilisation, several clinics are now exploring the serious possibility of replacing embryos at a later stage during development, usually the blastocyst stage. By doing this, they hope to exclude the transfer of embryos that would have had no chance of pregnancy, and thus improve the results of IVF.

8 Embryo transfer

When an embryo is ready to be put back into the uterus, it is put into a fine plastic tube together with a tiny drop of culture fluid. Usually two embryos, or occasionally three, are transferred together. After a brief vaginal examination the tube is inserted though the woman's cervix. The fluid containing the embryo or embryos is injected with extreme care into the uterus. Nearly all clinics will conduct the embryo transfer with the woman lying on her back. The procedure is very straightforward and so painless that it is usually not felt. Once the embryo transfer has taken place, the woman is usually required to remain lying down for ten to 30 minutes. It is thought that lying flat may help the embryo to 'stay put', but there is no good evidence for this. Indeed recent research strongly suggests that no amount of immediate movement will dislodge the embryo from its place in the uterus.

Some units have now adopted the practice we have been using at The Hammersmith Hospital for many years. Because it can be difficult to ensure that the catheter containing the embryos is in the right place inside the cavity of the woman, ultrasound is used. While the catheter is being inserted, an assistant places an ultrasound probe in the abdomen. The top of the catheter can be seen and the little blob of fluid containing the embryos can be placed in the cavity with certainty.

In good units, as soon as the transfer is completed, the catheter is handed back to the embryologist for checking. The catheter is examined under the microscope to make sure that there are no embryos sticking to it or remaining inside it. This is further evidence that the embryo transfer has been successful. If an embryo is left in the catheter, it is a simple matter to repeat the transfer procedure.

Hours or even days after embryo transfer nearly all women worry about moving around too vigorously. Many are so frightened of losing their embryos that they lie rigid in bed for hours at a time. This is quite unnecessary. In practice, it takes several days for an embryo to implant after it has been transferred to the uterus, and there is no evidence that routine activities have any effect on this process. If they did, then nobody would get pregnant. So women should not regard themselves as invalids, but for peace of mind it probably is a good idea to take things easy for a few days, staying away from work for a few days and avoiding sex for two weeks. It would certainly be wise not to travel abroad for a couple of weeks in order to stay in touch with the clinic.

9 Progesterone support

The early developing pregnancy requires the uterine lining to be in a suitable condition for implantation. Normally, when a pregnancy has occurred naturally, the ovary produces progesterone after ovulation and this stimulates the uterine lining to grow in the best possible way. In patients whose pituitary gland has been suppressed with Buserelin and other drugs, the ovary may not be capable of producing enough progesterone. For this reason it is common practice to give progesterone after an embryo transfer. There are a variety of ways of giving progesterone and different clinics may give it by different routes, and for differing periods of time. Many units give the initial doses of progesterone by injection for a few days and then this is followed by a vaginal pessary containing progesterone. This is easily absorbed through the vagina and acts on the uterine lining very satisfactorily. Most units continue this kind of treatment for between ten to fourteen days.

There is absolutely no advantage in continuing progesterone for longer than two weeks after transfer. Indeed continuing for longer than this may suppress onset of a period in a woman who is not pregnant.

Consequently the woman thinks she is pregnant simply because her uterine lining is incapable of bleeding. This a cruel deception, and to be avoided.

In a woman whose pituitary gland is not suppressed there is probably less reason to give progesterone. If the pituitary gland is not suppressed, then the ovary is perfectly capable of producing large amounts of progesterone, particularly if there have been several follicles in it before egg collection. In some units, however, an injection of HCG is given. This is probably quite unnecessary in most cases, but it will stimulate the punctured follicles to continue to produce progesterone.

10 Pregnancy testing

Everything up until this stage may have progressed smoothly with the embryos being transferred to the uterus without any difficulties. None the less, the chances are high that the woman will not get pregnant. Many embryos are lost before the menstrual period is due. They may have looked normal under a microscope, but it is likely that they were in some way poorly developed and incapable of producing a pregnancy. It should, however, be observed that many human embryos produced naturally during normal 'fertile' cycles are also incapable of subsequent development (see Figure 1.1).

Some clinics do not test for pregnancy at all; others suggest that the woman sends in a urine sample. At The Hammersmith Hospital we normally take blood samples on the twelfth or fourteenth day after embryo transfer – the earliest time at which a pregnancy can be detected. In some cases these hormone tests may be low, suggesting a pregnancy which is

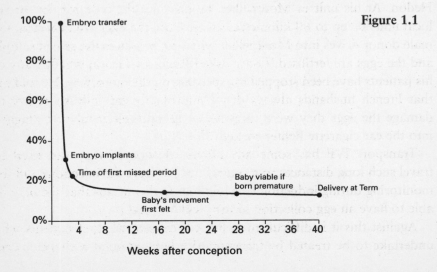

Figure 1.1

not implanting completely. If, after further testing, these hormones remain low, it suggests that the pregnancy is only 'biochemical', meaning that it is going to miscarry at a very early stage. Occasionally, a low test can mean that the pregnancy has implanted in a fallopian tube and is ectopic (see page 17). This will require further blood tests and ultrasound examinations in most cases. Conversely, a high level of pregnancy hormone human chorionic gonadotrophin suggests the possibility of twins – or a multiple pregnancy of some kind. This too will require a follow-up with ultrasound.

Transport IVF

One modification of IVF treatment which is somewhat in vogue is transport IVF. With this, eggs are collected in a local unit and sent to a central clinic for fertilisation and culture. The idea behind it is to cut down on the large costs involved in setting up a laboratory – though I have to say that the financial savings seem seldom to be passed on to the patient. Clinics offering transport IVF undertake to do the early part of the work. They conduct the stimulation of ovulation and the monitoring, and usually do an egg collection. Once the eggs are collected, these are normally sent in either the follicular fluid or culture medium, to a central IVF laboratory. The central laboratory is almost invariably in a major IVF unit. Embryo transfer is done at that unit after fertilisation with the partner's sperm has taken place.

The idea was first started in Paris, and probably the best example of transport IVF in Europe, is that run in France by Professor Bernard Hedon. At his unit in Montpellier, he provides the base for five or six local units or up to 60 kilometres away. Once the eggs are collected, the male donor drives into Montpellier where he produces the semen sample and the eggs are fertilised. I once asked Professor Hedon whether any of his patients have been stopped for speeding on the motorway. He told me that French husbands always drove improbably carefully so as not to damage the eggs they were carrying in the portable incubator, plugged into the car cigarette lighter socket.

Transport IVF has some advantages. A woman may not need to travel such long distances to a central unit, to have the injections and the monitoring during induction of ovulation. It also means that she may be able to have an egg collection in her local hospital.

Against this it is difficult to know, for certain, whether patients who undertake to be treated by transport IVF have as good a chance to get pregnant. My impression is that when all the treatment is done under one roof in a central unit, the results are distinctly better. Moreover, we frequently see patients who often have had poor information about what has happened to their eggs and embryos. Numerous patients who have had transport IVF feel that they have been unable to get definitive information about what has gone wrong during a particular treatment cycle. The division of responsibility between the local hospital and the central laboratory unit for patient communication is, I think, a significant drawback with transport IVF.

Trouble-shooting when a treatment has not worked after transport IVF is also more difficult. Because the local hospital generally does not have very sophisticated facilities, and may not do detailed hormone tests, the precise hormonal environment in which the follicles have developed may not be recorded. This makes assessment of the best line of action for a subsequent cycle of treatment very difficult. There is also sometimes a problem with lack of communication with patients once they get pregnant. For example, when the pregnancy hormone results indicate that an early miscarriage may be on the way, there are often problems getting good information from the local or central unit. Patients may not have access to the gynaecologist or clinician who was actually in charge of their care.

For what it is worth, my own feeling is that IVF treatment is generally better done in a large central unit. Even though it may be inconvenient to travel there and to spend time getting the treatment, the advantages of good quality information and better counselling seem to be really significant.

What are the real and perceived risks of IVF?

Abnormality of the baby

At the time of writing about 300,000 babies have been born around the world through IVF treatment, and there is no evidence to suggest that they are any more at risk from abnormalities than babies born after natural conception. Indeed, there is some evidence that after IVF certain types of abnormality (such as chromosome problems, for example Down's syndrome) are less common. IVF babies may tend to have more problems at birth, and stillbirths may be slightly more common, but this trend is not due to IVF itself but because women who conceive through IVF are more likely to be in the 'high-risk' group.

Ectopic pregnancy

IVF, rather surprisingly, can result in an ectopic pregnancy. If the tubes are damaged or partly blocked, this risk is greater, usually around two or three per cent. Although people often believe that IVF is a way of avoiding the risk of ectopic pregnancy, the incidence in women with damaged fallopian tubes after IVF is just as high as it is after tubal surgery. This is because after embryos have been placed in the uterus during transfer, one of them may leave it spontaneously and move into a fallopian tube, where it may implant. Even if the tubes have been totally removed, or blocked at the junction with the uterus, the risk of ectopic pregnancy is still present. This is because there is a small section of the tube in the wall of the uterus which cannot be removed or blocked off.

Multiple pregnancy

Women who have more than one embryo put into the uterus are more likely to have multiple pregnancy, with all the risks and complications that this causes. The British legal limit of a simultaneous transfer of three embryos per IVF cycle is a compromise between enhancing the chances of successful pregnancy and protecting against the risks of multiple pregnancy. In most clinics the chance of a twin pregnancy is about 25 per cent. Many infertile women after years of unsuccessful treatment are only too ready to accept such a risk, but while twins may not present too many problems, triplets are difficult to deal with and quadruplets can be disastrous. Quite apart from the risks of premature delivery and the risk of having an abnormal baby with brain damage, bringing up so many babies at once places a huge strain on a family.

Ovarian hyperstimulation (OHSS)

Drugs like FSH which stimulate the ovaries can cause the growth of too many follicles. This unwanted side-effect may occur because too much of the drug has been given, or it may occur because the ovaries are unusually sensitive. Over-reaction to ovulatory drugs is called ovarian hyperstimulation or ovarian hyperstimulation syndrome (OHSS).

Ovarian hyperstimulation is usually relatively mild, causing some swelling of the ovaries. There may be abdominal discomfort and feelings of being 'bloated'. Occasionally, there is pain low down in the pelvis. Mild hyperstimulation makes some women just feel unwell and it usually lasts for two or three days only. Such mild hyperstimulation occurs in as many as eight per cent of cycles.

Moderate hyperstimulation is associated with more pronounced discomfort in the abdomen, and sometimes general pelvic pain. The abdomen may be noticeably swollen and frequently people with this degree of hyperstimulation feel tired and breathless. In more pronounced cases there may be general fluid retention, including ankle swelling. Moderate hyperstimulation is relatively rare but when it occurs it may necessitate a short stay in hospital – usually just for rest and observation.

Severe hyperstimulation is rare in good units, and an event which we see only once in a few thousand cases. All the above symptoms are more pronounced. The breathlessness may be quite unpleasant and there may be a sufficient accumulation of fluid in the lung cavity or the abdomen to justify tapping it to drain it away. While the fluid is being retained in the wrong places, a woman may actually require an intravenous drip to give extra fluid into the bloodstream. This is because the loss of fluid into the tissues concentrates the blood and makes it thick. Hospital admission, which may be needed for a week or two, is essential because left untreated severe OHSS can cause quite serious illness.

Hyperstimulation always tends to be worse in pregnant women. It is also true that if you get OHSS after an embryo transfer and are pregnant, the pregnancy is more likely to stick. This is good news, but if OHSS is anticipated, most fertility units will take the sensible precaution of delaying the embryo transfer. In these circumstances it is good practice to freeze all embryos until there is no possible risk of harm by making the hyperstimulation worse. Once a new menstrual cycle has commenced, and the effect of all the drugs has gone, embryo transfer will be safe.

Nearly all moderate or severe cases of OHSS are preventable with adequate monitoring of ovarian development on ultrasound, though mild hyperstimulation is difficult to prevent. There are one or two conditions which predispose to OHSS, particularly polycystic ovary syndrome and some women just respond very briskly to superovulatory drugs. Careful assessment before an IVF treatment cycle will do much to avoid the more serious cases of hyperstimulation. Such women usually just require less FSH – with this precaution, and careful surveillance, they are quite safe.

Irregular periods

One of the complications associated with all of the drugs given during an IVF treatment cycle is that they can make the menstrual cycle irregular for a short time. It is quite common for the first natural period after a failed IVF treatment to come unexpectedly. The period may be early or late, and may last for longer than normal. It is uncommon for the period to be heavier than usual. On rare occasions menstrual irregularity may last for three or four months. If there are still problems after this, you should certainly see a gynaecologist for a check-up as these symptoms may be due not to the IVF, but some other medical cause.

Ovarian cancer

In recent years, there has been considerable worry that fertility drugs – the pills and injections used to induce ovulation – may cause cancer of the ovary. Most recently, this anxiety has been fanned by mostly well-meaning but sometimes irresponsible reports that doctors are not telling their patients the truth about the risks. In order to understand these risks, real or presumed, it is necessary to have some background.

Ovarian cancer is the sixth most common cancer in the world. In Britain, approximately fourteen women in every 100,000 are diagnosed in any given year (so roughly the chance of having it in any year is somewhat over 10,000 to one against). The incidence of ovarian cancer varies considerably from country to country – highest in Switzerland, about seventeen cases per 100,000 thousand to around one per 100,000 in parts of Africa and China. In some women there is an undoubted genetic tendency – it is more common in certain families. There is very limited evidence that the incidence of ovarian cancer has risen very slightly in some parts of the world, particularly Scandinavia, but in many other countries not at all.

Ovarian cancer is about twice as common in women who have not had children, compared with those who have had them. According to most studies it is also more common in women who have delayed child-bearing. Women who give birth before the age of 25 years old are less likely to get ovarian cancer and roughly speaking, with each five year delay after this the chance of getting ovarian cancer goes up by about ten per cent. Different studies show different associations with miscarriage – some reports suggest that if you have had a miscarriage, your chance of ovarian cancer is higher, but others suggest it may be lower.

Girls who start their periods before the age of eleven are at slightly greater risk of having ovarian cancer (perhaps one and a half times as much) as girls who start to menstruate after fifteen years old. Women who have an early menopause – before 45 years – are at lower risk than those who have their menopause after age 50. Taking the contraceptive pill seems protective – women who use the pill for longer than five years seem to reduce their risk of ovarian cancer by around 50 per cent. This effect may be greater in women who take the pill and who never have a child. It is unclear whether women on hormone replacement therapy (HRT) are at greater risk or not – probably not, though one study in Greece suggests that HRT may increase the risk by a factor of five times.

Infertile women are more likely – about twice as likely, overall – to develop ovarian cancer. Interestingly, this effect is also seen in women married to infertile men. One study in Israel by Dr Ron and his colleagues, in 1987, suggested that women married to infertile men may have as high as a six-fold chance of developing the disease – this has not been confirmed by other people. However, Dr Rossing and colleagues in the United States, in 1995, found that women with problems with ovulation had the highest risk. In Australia, Dr Venn and his colleagues have reported that unexplained infertility carried the biggest risk of ovarian cancer.

The most alarming study was that of Dr Whittemore and her colleagues in 1992, from the United States. They reported that there appeared to be a considerable increase in ovarian cancer in some women who had had FSH injections – Pergonal or Humegon – to treat infertility. It caused considerable anxiety and great controversy at the time, and it is this study which still alarms many people. Since it was published, the quality of this study has been heavily criticised. The number of women studied was small; there were very few clinical controls; there was no proper adjustment to allow for the fact that infertile women were at greater risk anyway; and there was no relation between the amount of drug given or the length of time it was given. Most important, probably the biggest flaw in the study was the fact that it was based on recall data – that is, that women with cancer were asked to remember whether they had ever taken fertility drugs. This is likely to introduce bias in reporting because there cannot be a proper control group for comparison.

Since that time there have been several studies and none clearly confirms the data presented by Whittemore. One Italian study by Dr Franceschi in 1994 suggested that there were actually fewer ovarian cancers in women who had taken these drugs. Another study from Canada reported similar findings. A Danish study in 1997 by Dr Mosgaard showed no overall risk, whilst an Israeli one by Dr Sushan suggested an extra risk of borderline tumours (a kind of pre-cancer) with stimulating drugs like HMG, but not frank, invasive cancer. There was no association with other fertility drugs given by injection.

David Healy and his colleagues in Australia are presently following up 30,000 women after IVF treatment. They published preliminary findings in October 1998. So far they have found no clear link between any of these drugs and cancer of the ovary. Moreover, their study has followed up women who have had as many as nine IVF cycles, and they have not found an increased risk of cancer or of borderline pre-cancers. Their impression is that women who have unexplained infertility may have an increased risk of ovarian cancer but that this is not related to the drugs they have been given but rather to the cause of the cancer.

In summary, then, there is no clear evidence of an increased risk of ovarian cancer in women having IVF treatment or those having fertility injections, compared with women who are infertile. There is some doubt about an increased risk in women who are given these drugs but who do not become pregnant. It seems that if you are infertile, but get successful treatment using these drugs, your risk of ovarian cancer falls. Possibly women who have unexplained infertility are at greater risk, but this is most likely to be due to a predisposing cause. The unexplained infertility in some of these women may occasionally be due to some ovarian abnormality – possibly some very early form of ovarian pre-cancer.

In Britain, these drugs in various forms have been used in many thousands of women since the 1960s. There has been no clear evidence that they cause ovarian cancer after what is now a very long time. Essentially, an injection of FSH is the injection of a hormone, which is normally produced by the body, and which is produced in very large amounts after the menopause. Few women are given these drugs for very long. We know that all infertility is associated with a slightly increased risk of cancer. Whilst I agree we should keep this matter under careful surveillance, I feel confident that we should continue to use these drugs. Indeed, by treating the infertility successfully, we may be reducing the risk of this disease. I would have no hesitation about giving them to my own family if needed.

Risks of other cancers

Cancer of the uterus is more common in women who have not had children. Cancer of the cervix is less common. There is absolutely no evidence that either cancer is caused by fertility drugs. Nor is there the slightest evidence that there is an increased risk of cancer of the breast. Dr Healy in Australia is following up the incidence of these diseases in his study as well and the findings to date are reassuring. Just as he found a small association between unexplained infertility, whether treated with fertility drugs or not, and ovarian cancer, so there was a similar increased incidence of uterine cancer in a few of these women.

This year there was one isolated report which suggested an increased risk of bowel cancer – based on a single case. I believe the way this report was written was shameful, because it was written in a manner that caused quite unnecessary alarm to a number of women. There is not the slightest evidence that drugs to induce ovulation, or IVF treatment, increase the risk of these cancers.

Premature menopause

A number of women undergoing IVF are worried that the drugs used to stimulate the ovaries may cause a premature menopause. Their worry is that, because so many eggs are being produced in one cycle, the ovary will run out sooner. There is no evidence in support of this view, and so far no evidence of premature menopause has been reported with these drugs.

Damage to ovarian vessels or surrounding structures

Although egg collection is done with great care under ultrasound control, the surgeon is looking only at an echo on what is effectively a computer screen. It is impossible to get a detailed image of the bowel, the bladder and small blood vessels. Inevitably, the advancing needle may hit one of these structures inadvertently as it enters the ovary.

Perforation of the bowel, I am sure, happens not infrequently after egg collection but is unnoticed by patient and doctor alike. It may occasionally account for unexplained pain after an egg collection because of inflammation around the perforation site. It is very unlikely to be dangerous. However, on rare occasions, patients can get an ovarian abscess, caused by infection or bacteria from the bowel leaking out of the hole caused by the needle. An abscess may form and this can on very rare occasions make a patient extremely ill. An open operation may exceptionally be needed to drain the infection site.

Very uncommonly, a blood vessel may be perforated. Excessive bleeding may be noticed by the surgeon, when the needle is withdrawn from the vagina. This normally stops, and is of no consequence. In fifteen years of experience of a large number of IVF cycles, I have known only two patients whose bleeding was sufficient to justify an open operation to secure the cut artery. This was easily done, and no serious damage resulted. After a blood transfusion, both patients made a healthy recovery.

Feelings during IVF treatment

Both men and women nearly always find IVF more stressful and emotionally demanding than they expected. Regular attendance at hospital, the inevitable waiting around, travelling and staying away from home are all tiring. The monitoring of follicle growth and the build-up to egg collection are particular occasions of tension and worry. As we have seen, often a man may find it difficult under this kind of pressure to produce his semen when it is needed. Women who are in a job invariably wonder how they are going to cope with work, travelling and waiting at hospital, and also what they will tell their employers. In fact, generally employers are far more forgiving than most women expect. It is also true that it usually possible to cope with one's job whilst undergoing IVF. Flexibility of hours is helpful, but in reality the only days off which are really necessary are the day of egg collection and the day of transfer. We have not found there to be an improved pregnancy rate in women who stop work. The only reason for considering stopping work is simply to reduce your level of stress. This may make you feel better, but will not affect success or failure of treatment.

IVF is very like being in a steeplechase – once on, you can not generally get off, and there are unexpected and sometimes unpleasant bumps, if not actual falls. Waiting to see if the follicles respond to drugs is a critical hurdle. The egg collection is a major fence and the approach to it is usually a time of anxiety. People are often disappointed because they feel they have produced too few eggs. It is fairly devastating to wake from an egg collection to find that only one, or even no egg at all has been collected. Then there is the two or three day wait to see if fertilisation and embryo development has happened. This period of time is often tense and people frequently feel restless, or have vivid dreams.

Once the embryo has been put back in the uterus, the tension is if anything generally more difficult. For women undergoing IVF this will usually be the first time they have clearly had the experience of knowing they have produced an embryo. Most patients fantasise that they are pregnant once the embryo transfer has been done; a very difficult emotion with which to cope, given that 80 per cent of the time a normal menstrual period is just around the corner. Nearly all women start to believe they feel as if they might be pregnant – or alternatively as if they have lost the pregnancy – when in fact these feelings are only symptomatic of the general turmoil this treatment sometimes brings.

The couple must wait to see if the embryo has successfully implanted, this time with no medical procedures to distract them from their worries. Sometimes when the menstrual period comes, it comes late. It may just be after a delay of a few days or so, but if it is as long as a week (perhaps with an equivocal or borderline pregnancy test) the disappointment that follows its arrival can be all-consuming.

Even after the embryo has implanted, there is still the risk of miscarriage. This is such a devastating experience in normal circumstances, that little effort is required to imagine how cruel it must seem to an infertile couple who have already experienced such an uphill struggle to conceive in the first place. On top of the grief they will feel for the loss of their baby, they may well feel a profound sense of despair. The prospect of having to pick themselves up and start all over again may seem overwhelming.

The loss will inevitably bring home to them the fact of their infertility, with all the attendant feelings of inadequacy, guilt and worthlessness. Recrimination between partners and towards the doctors responsible for their treatment often occurs. Couples may also feel a tremendous sense of isolation with this latest setback to their hopes of taking part with normal social contacts with people of their age group and all the talk of babies, children and schools. Their feelings of jealousy may be intense, and the woman's visits to hospital, where other women are attending for antenatal care, may seem unbearable.

Often the woman's grief for the lost pregnancy will be followed by depression. She may lose all confidence in herself and find herself crying frequently. She may feel lethargic and unable to concentrate or to derive any pleasure from activities she normally enjoys. She may lose her appetite and find it difficult to sleep. She feels helpless in face of the simplest daily tasks.

The brunt of a lost pregnancy is borne inevitably by the woman, but it is sometimes forgotten how difficult it can also be for the man. He is likely to be deeply upset by the physical distress his partner will have endured, and, in seeking to give her the emotional support she needs, may bury his own feelings of grief.

These ups and downs are an inevitable fact of much IVF treatment. Nevertheless, it would be quite misleading for me to be too negative about how people feel during these treatments. Very many people find it an extremely positive experience. Indeed it is very often the case that couples find it far less unpleasant or demanding, than they expected. Women quite frequently find it easier to cope with a second or subsequent cycle, once they know what to expect. Very often infertile couples feel they are doing something definitive which will resolve their problem of infertility, and how they approach it. For so many women and men it is undoubtedly better to have gone through IVF and failed, than not to have attempted it all.

2
Tests before infertility treatment

When to test for infertility

Throughout this book, I emphasise the need for adequate diagnostic investigation. It is so important to know why conception is not taking place, not least because that in itself can bring considerable comfort to couples who are finding treatment difficult to tolerate. It goes without saying that the key to the best and most successful treatment is to try, if at all possible, to clearly establish what is causing the infertility.

On average, it takes most couples at least five months to conceive normally. It is perfectly usual to take up to a year to conceive. Testing is needed only after this period unless there are earlier indications that there may be a problem. Women much over thirty years old are likely to be less fertile and may take longer to get pregnant. Consequently, although there may be little wrong, they may wish to be investigated sooner.

These are the other circumstances when it may be advisable to seek advice from a specialist and probably earlier investigation:

In women

History/symptoms	Possible cause/result
No periods for some time	Probably not ovulating
Very infrequent periods	Not ovulating regularly
Painful periods or deep pain on sex	Inflammation or endometriosis
Recently increasingly heavy periods	Problems in the uterus, possibly fibroids
Operations (e.g. biopsy) on the cervix	Abnormal cervical cells
Previous operation for ovarian cyst	Adhesions or tubal problem
Previous burst appendix	Tubal problems
Previous problems with contraceptive coil	Adhesions or tubal blockage
Infection after pregnancy or labour	Pelvic inflammation

In men

History/symptoms	Possible cause/result
Mumps during adult life	Poor sperm production
Testicle injury	Poor sperm production
Previous undescended testicle	Poor/absent sperm
Previous hernia operation	Damage to testicular tubes
Past inflammation of testes	Sperm antibodies/ poor sperm
Inflammation of prostate gland	Poor sperm motility
Heavy smoking or alcohol	Poor sperm motility

Prompt diagnosis

Once a couple have decided to seek infertility tests a diagnosis should usually be reached within six months. It is important that a thorough range of tests be undertaken. Often a cause is found halfway through testing and treatment is started without any further tests, although there may well be more than one cause of infertility. This premature diagnosis can lead to a delay in getting effective treatment.

It is well worth making yourself as familiar with the various tests as you can. Even experienced specialists may occasionally forget to perform an important test and might benefit from a reminder. If you find this difficult, discuss your case with your family doctor. He will probably have made the original referral and his role is above all to keep an eye on your general care. Do not hesitate to tell your doctor if you think tests are taking too long or are not being done. He can often speed up the process dramatically by outlining your various concerns in a letter. The specialist, whose practice depends on satisfying patients sent by family doctors, will seldom take offence.

While your family doctor may be in a position to do some simple tests – like a sperm count – most will send their infertile patients to a specialist. If you have a particular clinic or specialist in mind, you can ask your doctor to refer you accordingly. For the first visit it is generally best, I think, if the couple attend together. Hospitals can be forbidding places and it is good for morale to share what may be a stressful experience.

The first appointment

The specialist will want to know how old the couple are and how long they have been trying to conceive. He or she will inquire into the history of any previous pregnancies.

Some women worry that they may be asked about a previous pregnancy about which their partner has no knowledge. If it is impossible to be candid during the joint visit, they should arrange to see the specialist alone on a separate occasion. Doctors will not reveal such private information to anyone else, including a partner.

The specialist will want to know the woman's gynaecological history and the frequency of recent menstrual periods. He or she may also inquire about how often the couple have sexual intercourse. Some couples may find such questions embarrassing, but they are obviously relevant.

A consultant may conduct an internal examination, although provided a woman is having regular intercourse and there is no history suggesting uterine abnormalities or an ovarian cyst, it usually provides very little information. It is also an examination which can easily be deferred until a later visit when confidence has been gained if a woman is especially anxious or embarrassed. Examination of the man also often gives only limited information, unless he is known to have an abnormal sperm count. Even then examination of most male patients usually reveals little detectable abnormality. Occasionally a damaged testis may be smaller than normal, or there may be cysts or abnormal swelling which will require special tests.

Tests for the man

Sperm count

One normal sperm count is not by itself an indication of a man being fully fertile. There may be problems which cannot be detected on a routine count. On the other hand, one abnormal or low count does not necessarily mean that there is anything wrong. Most men produce poor quality semen from time to time, especially if they have had a recent illness or have been under stress. Good clinics will therefore assess a man's fertility on the basis of several sperm counts and usually do specialised sperm function tests as well.

For a routine count, semen should be delivered to the clinic within two hours of its collection. The clinic will provide a small pot with a form asking a few basic details. Most men prefer to produce semen by masturbation; some like their partners to help them or find it easier to interrupt intercourse and ejaculate into the pot. It can be difficult to get all the semen into the pot, and an incomplete sample may make the count abnormally low. Sperm function tests generally require freshly ejaculated semen. Clinics doing such tests will provide premises for a man to produce sperm in comfortable surroundings.

A routine sperm count includes the following tests:

Semen volume. An ejaculate is normally about two–five millilitres (up to a teaspoonful). If the volume is less than this, the man may not be producing enough secretions, or part of the sample may not have been collected at ejaculation.

Sperm numbers. Normally there are more than 40 million in each millilitre. There may be a problem if there are fewer than 20 million, but a few men are fully fertile even when they produce only 2 or 3 million sperm per millilitre of semen.

Sperm motility. At least 40 per cent of the sperm should be moving.

Normal sperm. At least 65 per cent of the sperm should look normal under a microscope. If there are a lot of abnormal sperm, it may mean that there is a problem with their manufacture in the testicles.

'Clumping' bacteria, white blood cells. A good laboratory will observe whether any sperm have stuck together. 'Clumping' may indicate infection, or possibly antibodies to the sperm.

Antibodies. Some laboratories do specific test for antibodies attacking the sperm. Antibodies are produced by some response to injury or infection. These are usually produced as a part of the body's defence system. However, when they attack the sperm they can prevent them working normally.

A good clinic will not generally give the result of sperm tests over the telephone. They will want to be sure of who they are talking to, and to be able to provide proper emotional support if it is needed. It is a good thing, if possible, for partners to go together to get the test result. It is an important time for both of them, and it can be a heavy burden for a woman to go to the clinic by herself to find that her partner has a problem.

Sperm function tests

Sperm function tests are more detailed and complex assessments of male fertility. They vary somewhat from clinic to clinic. Very often, they include a detailed computerised analysis of the way sperm swims. This can be a very useful prediction of the likelihood of fertilisation, where *in vitro* fertilisation (IVF) is to be used. Another very common sperm function test is to place the sperm in particular culture solutions, usually the culture media which are used during IVF. After a period of time assessments can then be made to see how far the sperm have swum in the culture, and to see how mobile they are after a period of time outside the body.

Other assessments of sperm can be made by more detailed examination, such as detailed microscopy. Some specialised units examine individual sperm under exceptionally high magnification, using an electron microscope. This can be a source of important information about the kind of abnormalities which are present in individual sperm and may occasionally be used before IVF.

Sperm culture

If there is evidence of an infection, some laboratories culture the semen to try to identify the bacterium responsible as a preliminary to antibiotic treatment. But these cultures tend to be unreliable.

Fructose measurement

If there are no sperm in the semen, this may be because there is a blockage either above or below the seminal vesicles. The seminal vesicles produce fructose, a simple sugar which is easily measured in the semen. If the semen is low in fructose, this suggests that the blockage is below the seminal vesicles, which helps to direct a surgeon where to look.

Split ejaculate test

During ejaculation, the first part of the semen tends to be richer in sperm even when the sperm count is low. The split ejaculate test helps to evaluate whether this 'concentrated' semen may be worth collecting for artificial insemination.

Human zona penetration and attachment tests

To test the ability of a sperm to penetrate the zona ('shell') of the egg the sperm can be mixed with dead human eggs. This is a largely experimental procedure, at present available in only a few research centres.

Another similar test involves counting the number of sperm which attach themselves to the zona (the stage in fertilisation just before penetration of the zona itself occurs). This is also experimental, but it is promising and has provided some useful information about sperm function.

The post-coital test

This test usually takes place between six and 36 hours after sexual intercourse. It gives very limited information about the ability of the sperm to survive for a longer period of time. The specialist takes a fluid sample from the woman's cervix during an internal examination, which will feel like a cervical smear test. He or she then immediately examines the cervical mucus under a microscope to see if there are any sperm present and whether they are moving around.

This test needs to be performed during the first half of the woman's menstrual cycle, just before ovulation when the mucus is most easily penetrated by the sperm. It may help the specialist to assess not only the man's fertility but also whether the woman is ovulating normally and has a healthy cervix.

There are so many reasons why a post-coital test may be negative that this test is less relevant than it used to be. Many clinics and specialists have abandoned it completely.

Hormone tests

Some men, particularly those whose testes are no longer capable of producing sperm properly, may have abnormal hormone tests. Most important of these tests is one to detect the presence of a raised level of follicle stimulating hormone (FSH). Follicle stimulating hormone is normally produced by the pituitary gland at the base of the brain. This hormone is usually a stimulus to the testes and tells them to manufacture sperm. If for some reason the testes are unable to produce sperm, then the brain encourages the production of more FSH. Consequently, a very high level of FSH suggest that the testicle is no longer able to respond to the brain's message and that sperm manufacture in the testis – spermatogenesis – is failing or has failed completely. High levels of FSH are often an indication that there will be no viable sperm in the ejaculate, or even in the testes themselves. It is a particularly useful test for those men who may be trying to decide whether or not to undergo one of the more complicated procedures associated with IVF, particularly sperm microinjection (see page 66), or recovery of sperm from the testes. It is important to realise that most men with high FSH levels, although they may have a degree of testicular failure, are producing completely normal amounts of male hormone (testosterone). In this type of infertility, therefore, although there may be testicular failure, there will not be any other problems with sexuality or virility.

On rare occasions a man may be producing insufficient FSH. This is usually because the pituitary gland has been damaged in some way. Alternatively, that part of the brain which regulates the pituitary gland may be damaged. In many such cases, administration of this hormone is all that is required to get a man to produce normal sperm. Nevertheless, it must be emphasised that the conditions which cause a deficiency of FSH are really very rare.

Testicular biopsy

A testicular biopsy is where a surgeon takes a small piece of tissue from the testes itself. The piece of tissue is then prepared and examined under a microscope. Microscopic evaluation can be used to determine whether the testes is capable of producing sperm in the normal way. It may also be used to see if there are any normal, viable sperm which might be used for one of the more advanced IVF procedures. Sometimes the testicular biopsy can be frozen so that the sperm inside it may be used at a later date for fertilising the eggs of the man's partner, after IVF treatment (see page 105).

Testicular biopsy is usually performed under a general anaesthetic and sometimes can be done as a day case in hospital. Very occasionally, the patient may need to stay in hospital overnight after this procedure. Commonly the biopsy is taken out of a small incision in the scrotum which requires a couple of small stitches.

Thermography

This test, which is nowadays done only occasionally, measures the temperature of the testes. Sometimes men with low sperm counts and very prominent veins in the testicles – so-called varicocoeles – may have somewhat overheated testes. This test is of limited value, as it is by no sure that overheating is the key problem.

Ultrasound

From time to time a doctor may order an ultrasound examination of the testes. This is a completely painless operation which can be done on an outpatient basis. The ultrasound probe is placed on the scrotum, and an image of the testes can be seen on the computer screen. Small cysts or very occasionally tumours in the testes may be identified by this method. Sometimes the presence of such abnormalities indicates that the tubes from the testes are blocked, or that the testes are not capable of producing sperm in the normal amounts in the normal way.

Chromosome (karyotype) testing

Some men who are not producing enough normal sperm, or who are hardly producing any sperm at all, may have a genetic abnormality. Most commonly this is a chromosomal abnormality which affects the male, Y chromosome. One chromosomal abnormality which occurs occasionally is a 'translocation', when parts of two separate chromosomes are stuck together. In the case of either of these abnormalities, it is quite common to find that a man is sub-fertile, usually because his sperm are incapable of fertilising or because there are insufficient sperm coming out of the testes.

Chromosome testing involves a blood test. Once the blood has been collected, it is cultured for between two–four weeks. After staining of individual white blood cells, an assessment of the chromosomes can be made. This test is valuable not only for various causes of male infertility, but some causes of unexplained fertility. Unfortunately, chromosome tests are not capable of detecting all genetic abnormalites causing poor sperm production.

Tests for the woman

Ovulation
Good clinics employ more than one test for ovulation.

Blood test for progesterone. This is the most widely used test for ovulation, although it provides only indirect evidence that ovulation has taken place. Progesterone is one of the female hormones that the ovary produces during the second half of a woman's cycle. The blood test measures the amount of progesterone the ovary produces, although it cannot detect whether an egg has actually left the ovary. In Britain this hormone measurement is usually expressed as 'nmol (nanomols) per litre', and in America as 'ng (nanograms) per litre'. The normal level after ovulation is 30nmol per litre (10ng per litre).

The level of progesterone is at its highest about a week after ovulation and is maintained for three to five days. It is therefore usual to take a blood test on the twenty-first day of the menstrual cycle. It may be helpful to repeat it two or three days later to confirm that the rise is maintained. The level falls sharply immediately before a period, so a test taken within a day or two of bleeding may be meaningless. Many couples become discouraged when they have a low reading, but it may simply mean that the first day of the period occurred sooner or later than expected.

Temperature charting. This is not strictly an 'essential' test. I include it here because a few clinics place considerable importance on temperature charts, and they can provide a limited indication of whether ovulation is occurring. They also have the advantage of involving a simple procedure which the woman can administer herself.

While it is true that a woman's body temperature rises slightly after ovulation (probably because the higher level of progesterone increases her metabolism) many normally ovulating women have no discernible change. Much needless distress is caused by perfectly fertile women charting their temperatures in this way. On the other hand, some women who are not ovulating may none the less notice a rise in temperature after the mid-cycle and wrongly conclude that their ovaries are working properly.

Some women believe that their temperature chart will tell them when they are at their most fertile and use it to time intercourse. The evidence for the value of this approach is limited.

Kits from the chemist. A popular method of testing for ovulation is the use of luteinising hormone (LH) kits which can be bought over the counter in most chemist's shops. These are dipped in the first specimen of urine passed each morning and are able to detect when there is a marked increase in the level of the hormone LH. As the follicle matures in the ovary and the time for ovulation draws closer, the follicle produces increase amounts of oestrogen. This gets into the blood stream, circulates to the brain and tells the pituitary gland to secrete LH – the message to the ovary to ovulate because the egg in the follicle is close to maturity.

LH kits are a good idea in theory, but there are a number of problems associated with them which makes them only of limited value. Firstly, they only test for the sudden surge of LH which should occur about 36 hours before ovulation. Some women have an abnormal surge but are still ovulating. Other women, particularly those in the older age group and women with polycystic ovaries, may produce high levels of LH which are not associated with ovulation, at the wrong time during the menstrual cycle. This confuses the test hopelessly. In other women the test just doesn't seem to work properly. But whatever the reason for using these kits they certainly add to the strain of infertility, because they encourage people to time intercourse. This domination of one's sex life can make infertility an ever more demanding and emotional experience. Finally these kits are not cheap, costing about £25 each month.

Endometrial biopsy

An endometrial biopsy can be performed during the second half of the woman's menstrual cycle. It involves removing a small piece of the uterine lining (the endometrium) and examining it under the microscope. In this way it can be determined whether the uterine lining has been exposed and has responded to the progesterone that is normally produced by the ovary after ovulation.

The best time for an endometrial biopsy is between the eighteenth and twenty-eighth day of a twenty-eight-day cycle up to the time of menstruation. The cervix is cleaned after a simple examination and a small pipe is inserted through it. A tiny scraping of the uterine lining is quickly removed. It can cause brief discomfort – a small cramp-like period pain. Because some women are nervous about the pain that can occasionally occur many clinics delay this test until the patient comes for laparoscopy under anaesthesia (see page 37).

In recent years the endometrial biopsy has been used increasingly to look for biochemical markers which may indicate whether the lining of the uterus is developing properly. These biochemical markers may be particularly valuable in ascertaining whether or not the embryo is capable of implanting in the uterus. While it is expected that assessments of these biochemical markers may be extremely valuable in the future, so far they are only of experimental use. None the less, this is one of the areas of infertility investigation which shows considerable promise.

Ovarian ultrasound

Ultrasound tests uses high frequency sound waves which are passed through the body. When the sound waves hit tissue an echo is given off. These are then picked up and analysed by a computer displayed on a TV monitor. Ultrasound allows measurement of structures inside the abdomen. In the case of ovarian ultrasound, the waves are aimed at the ovaries through the abdominal wall or the vagina. These lie just behind the bladder, and because water is a good conductor of sound, the best pictures may be obtained when the bladder is full. The woman will therefore be asked to drink some water before an abdominal ultrasound is carried out. Nearly all IVF centres now use vaginal ultrasound with a small ultrasound probe into the vagina. This has the advantage of avoiding the discomfort of a full bladder and gives better quality images than those obtained using a probe on the abdomen.

The ultrasound machine can determine whether the follicles are growing properly and when they have ruptured – that is, when a woman has ovulated. It is also very useful for detecting polycystic ovaries (see page 35) and early pregnancy. Ultrasound is very valuable for detecting cysts and ovarian damage due to endometriosis. It can help in assessment of the uterus – particularly fibroids – but generally X-rays or magnetic resonance imaging (MRI) (page 36) are rather more detailed and accurate.

Hormone profiles

The levels of hormones in blood can be measured during the early part of a menstrual cycle, thereby helping to pinpoint a hormone abnormality which may be affecting ovulation. Measurement of the hormones oestrogen, LH and FSH are the most valuable.

On very rare occasions, low levels of FSH and LH may be found. These may indicate the need for hormone treatment. Much more usual are raised levels, which commonly indicate polycystic ovaries. High levels of FSH are unfortunately a sign that the ovaries may not have many eggs left in them. Sadly women with high levels of FSH (much over 10 international units [the standard recognised measurement] and therefore with a degree of ovarian failure) may have great difficulty in producing good eggs. Raised levels of testosterone (which women also produce normally) suggest that ovulation is not taking place normally. This is sometimes seen with certain types of polycystic ovary syndrome.

The hormone prolactin which is produced by the pituitary gland may also be raised. Some women are worried that they have a high prolactin level, but if their periods are regular and if progesterone levels are normal and consistent with ovulation, then this is irrelevant. More commonly high prolactin levels are an indication that there may be polycystic ovaries.

Testing the fallopian tubes and the uterus

The hysterosalpingogram (HSG). The hysterosalpingogram (HSG) is an X-ray of the uterus and fallopian tubes. It is an unduly neglected test that some doctors believe has been superseded by telescopic inspection under anaesthetic. In fact, it provides information which it is impossible to get in any other way. Moreover, it is an easy test to do and less expensive than those requiring anaesthesia.

A little dye is placed in the uterus and X-rays are taken during an injection, revealing whether the tubes are open or not. The quality of the shadow on the X-ray can give a very good outline of the inside of the uterus, and the shadows which the tubes themselves produce give a good indication of the existence of tubal blockage and whether there is any extensive scarring. With very modern X-ray equipment – especially using digital enhancement – great detail can be revealed and invaluable information obtained.

At The Hammersmith Hospital we usually organise an HSG as soon as possible after the first visit to the clinic if this has not been previously done. By the time the couple return for their follow-up appointment we will have a detailed assessment of the quality of the tubes and the uterus.

The X-ray is done following a simple internal examination. The doctor inserts a thin tube through the cervix. The instrument that fits inside the cervix is no larger than a ball-point pen refill. A small amount of dye is injected into the uterus, and its progress is monitored on a television screen. About six X-rays may be taken. The whole procedure takes about ten minutes. With digital enhancing equipment, a conventional X-ray film is unnecessary. Increasingly a computer image is used which makes the whole procedure simpler for the patient and more informative for the specialists.

HSG used to have a reputation for causing discomfort, but this is now completely unjustified. Most women in our hospital do not even realise that the test has started or finished. Sometimes the insertion of the tube can cause a little discomfort, but it is no worse than a period pain. Persistent pain after the HSG can indicate infection and is not normal. Any woman who experiences this should contact the hospital no matter how late at night it might be.

HSG is very good at revealing adhesions inside the uterus, as well as fibroids, scarring of the uterine muscle and polyps. It can also reveal congenital abnormalities of the uterus which are a not uncommon cause of infertility. In the area where the tubes join the uterus, the internal plumbing is extremely delicate and small. The HSG reveals far more effectively than a laparoscopy whether there is any scar tissue here or polyps in the tube itself. A good X-ray also clearly reveals any scarring in the tubal lining and its folds.

At The Hammersmith Hospital we have many patients coming to us who have undergone IVF unsuccessfully in other clinics. All too frequently we find that an HSG has not been done, or has been done inadequately. When the investigation is performed properly, we commonly uncover a clear reason for the failure of the earlier IVF attempts. As most of these contributing factors are entirely correctable, it is a great pity that more emphasis is not placed on getting good quality X-rays before IVF treatment is considered.

Magnetic resonance imaging (MRI). Magnetic resonance imaging (sometimes called nuclear magnetic resonance) is a recently developed technique for investigating the pelvic organs which can provide extremely valuable information. In particular, it can provide evidence of damage to the wall of the uterus and scar tissue in the muscle. We frequently use it when we suspect that the patient has the condition called adenomyosis, which is where the lining of the womb – the endometrium – grows into the wall of the uterus. This is a frequent cause of infertility and may also cause painful periods. It is quite common in older women who have been unsuccessful with IVF.

In order to get a magnetic resonance image, the part of the body to be examined has to be placed in an intense magnetic field. This is produced by a large coil which totally surrounds the body. It is a totally painless procedure which causes no discomfort of any kind. Moreover, because it does not use X radiation, it is entirely risk free. It can, however, be a slightly unnerving experience. This is because the machine itself makes a considerable noise while it is in operation and because the patient lying inside the coil may have to keep still for several minutes at a time. With the latest equipment, MRI can give images of very high quality, far better than those achieved, for example, using ultrasound.

Because MRI is a relatively expensive test, it is not employed routinely. At The Hammersmith Hospital, we use this test only when we have a high suspicion that the uterine wall may be abnormal, generally in patients who have also failed IVF. Patients who have slightly irregular but chronically painful periods and some patients who bleed during the menstrual cycle are rather more likely to have adenomyosis and it is generally in the case of these women that this test is most useful.

Laparoscopy

Laparoscopy is by far the most important test for female infertility. In my view it nearly always should be considered before entering an IVF programme, unless it is clearly known that a woman has no fallopian tubes, or that there is no possibility of corrective surgery.

A thin telescope is inserted into the abdominal cavity through a small hole made in the navel. Carbon dioxide, which has previously been passed into the abdomen, separates the organs so that they can be seen more easily. The telescope is no thicker than a fountain pen, but with the improvement in modern optics enables photographs of superb quality to be taken. A surgeon can use the laparoscope to inspect the outside of the uterus, and to test the tubes to see if they are open by injecting coloured dye through them.

Laparoscopy is best performed during the second half of the woman's cycle, because then a surgeon can examine the ovaries for signs of ovulation, and because a piece of the lining of the uterus can be taken to see if it is likely to be receptive to a fertilised egg. Some infertility centres perform a laparoscopy under a local anaesthetic as a day-care procedure.

But a general anaesthetic is more usual. The laparoscopy itself takes about 20 to 40 minutes and carries no serious risk. Recovery is rapid and most women can go home within four to six hours of the procedure.

Afterwards the patient will normally find two small dressings on the abdomen. One covers a single stitch in the navel, and the other a tiny hole near the pubic hairline. This second hole is used to place any fine probes the thickness of a small knitting needle into the abdominal cavity which may be required to get a better view.

Laparoscopy usually causes very little pain or discomfort although some women may feel unwell and need to rest in bed for twenty-four hours. The commonest side-effects are:

- Soreness in the abdomen.
- Soreness in one or other shoulder. This is because the carbon dioxide injected into the abdomen can irritate the nerves to the abdominal lining which happen also to supply the shoulder area.
- Vaginal bleeding. This may occur if the surgeon manipulates the cervix during injection of the dye to check the tubes. It may last two or three days and sometimes longer.
- A sore throat. This rarely lasts more than 24 hours and results from the tube which the anaesthetist has placed down the throat to ensure a safe anaesthetic.
- Sleeplessness or vivid dreams the night after. This is frequently experienced by anyone who has had a general anaesthetic.
- Sickness due to the anaesthetic. Few people experience this nowadays because the action of the drugs is more gentle than it once was. There are special drugs which can be given to people known to be prone to sickness after anaesthesia.

The benefits of a laparoscopy are considerable:

- It is the best way to determine whether the tubes have been damaged.
- It shows up adhesions in the abdominal cavity very clearly.
- It gives a direct view of the ovaries, and, if it is performed in the second half of the woman's cycle, enables the surgeon to see whether there has been recent ovulation.
- It gives a good idea of the size of the ovaries. This is important because women with very small ovaries are more likely to produce few eggs during stimulation for IVF.
- It is the best way to detect endometriosis.
- It gives an excellent view of the outside of the uterus and may help to detect fibroids or a congenital problem in the womb.

- It helps to detect diseases in the abdominal cavity or in the ovaries.
- After laparoscopy more women immediately conceive than would be expected by chance. About fifteen per cent of our patients with open tubes conceive within three months of laparoscopy.

Hysteroscopy

This test is usually performed under a quick general anaesthetic on a day visit to the hospital. A small telescope, called an hysteroscope, is passed into the uterus through the vagina. It is an excellent means of detecting any polyps, uterine fibroids, adhesions or congenital abnormalities which may be suspected following the results of an HSG test. It can also be used to treat some of these conditions by guiding instruments inside the uterus. It does not replace the HSG which gives detailed information of a different kind.

Tuboscopy and falloposcopy

Tuboscopy requires a fine telescope to be inserted through the abdominal wall under general anaesthetic, in order to inspect the inside of the ovarian end of the fallopian tube. This test, which can be combined with laparoscopy, is of only limited value, except to the surgeon who can charge large fees for it. One alternative is a falloscopy, namely the passage of a very fine telescope into the fallopian tube from below, through the vagina and uterus. This telescope is about the thickness of a piece of linen thread, and gives a view of the uterine end of the tube. It is usually attached to a television camera and the result viewed on a screen, but because the optic fibre is so narrow the resolution of the picture is not as good as that seen using tuboscopy. It probably has even less value than tuboscopy and is only included here for completeness.

Karyotype (chromosome) test

Just as men may have a problem with their chromosomes causing abnormal production of sperm, so too can a chromosome problem cause infertility in women. Some women who are not ovulating at all have a chromosome abnormality, but it is now well known that women who are having repeated miscarriages, and some women who are not getting pregnant at all, can have a variety of chromosome abnormalities. If a chromosomal abnormality is suspected, this can be detected using blood tests. After culturing the white cells in the blood for three to four weeks, the individual chromosomes in the cell can be counted and identified.

Until recently chromosome abnormalities were totally untreatable. However, some infertile women (particularly those who miscarry frequently) have a chromosomal abnormality which may be screened for in their embryos. Under these circumstances preimplantation genetic diagnosis (PGD) (page 83) can sometimes be used and may help them to achieve a normal pregnancy. When a chromosome abnormality cannot be treated at all, egg donation from a normal donor may be the only alternative possibility.

IVF should ideally be contemplated only when a further attempt at making a diagnosis for the infertility has been done first. Unfortunately, because IVF is seen so frequently as a panacea for infertility treatment, far too many men and women attempt this treatment when it could be that other, simpler, less expensive treatments might be more applicable. It is of course true that sometimes a cause for the infertility cannot be found. Under these circumstances IVF may be useful. Carefully performed IVF, particularly in a well-established and large unit, is very likely to give an understanding as to the underlying cause of infertility. IVF may also result in a successful pregnancy and consequently the immediate concern about having a baby is solved.

Dilation and curettage (D & C)

Some women who are having difficulty conceiving are still brought into hospital for a 'womb scrape'. It does no harm, but is generally useless unless it is done at the time of a laparoscopy; then an endometrial biopsy may give limited information about the state of the uterine lining. It is frequently performed in the vain belief that it makes it easier to conceive.

Measurement of trace elements, vitamins, hair testing

I cannot emphasise enough how strongly I feel about these tests which are, almost certainly, a confidence trick. Some private clinics prey on the desperation of infertile couples by offering these tests of no obvious value. A typical clinic may charge considerable sums to examine a lock of hair for trace elements. The result may show an absence of zinc, magnesium, cadmium, vitamins or some other substances which have absolutely no proved relevance to human fertility.

3
Other forms of assisted reproduction

As outlined in earlier chapters, *in vitro* fertilisation (IVF) is most complicated and generally expensive; frequently there are other more appropriate treatments for infertility. This chapter describes other forms of assisted reproduction and routine infertility treatment, what they are and when to do them.

Artificial insemination

Artificial insemination (AI) is the process by which sperm are injected either into the vagina, cervix or more usually, the uterus, near the time of ovulation. It is done when sperm donation is needed. Insemination with one's partner's semen, known as 'artificial insemination by husband' (AIH), is also used frequently. AI is best done by direct injection into the uterus (intra-uterine insemination or IUI). This improves the chance of sperm getting into the fallopian tubes, where fertilisation normally occurs.

Vaginal or cervical insemination

Semen is injected directly into the vagina through a small tube and may be deliberately placed in the cervix. The woman lies with her knees up for a few minutes, but insemination causes no discomfort. This may be used for basic routine insemination but is indicated in some couples who are having difficulties with sex or if there is an anatomical problem with the cervix preventing the sperm getting to the right place.

This treatment has little point for men with low sperm counts because normal intercourse will allow sperm to be introduced into the cervical canal. One advantage of AIH is that insemination can be timed to take place just before ovulation. However, this advantage is not much counterbalanced by the invasion of privacy it involves, as it does not always greatly improve the chance of pregnancy.

Intrauterine insemination (IUI)

The sperm must undergo special preparation before IUI. They may be 'washed', i.e. repeatedly mixed in special fluid (or media), and then spun in a tube that removes débris. They may be separated by the 'swim' process, whereby the sperm are placed at the bottom of a tube of medium and healthy sperm may swim up to the surface where they are collected by suction through a glass tube. Injecting neat, unwashed semen into the uterus is dangerous because it can cause allergic reactions.

These methods may be used if there are large numbers of dead sperm or cells in the semen. No concentration takes place, just purification. They may also be used if there are sperm antibodies, as washing may occasionally get rid of them.

IUI can be a little uncomfortable, but shouldn't cause pain. It is most effective when the ovaries are stimulated by either clomiphene tablets or injections of Follicle Stimulating Hormone (FSH). This results in more than one egg being produced. Stimulation of egg production must be gentle because of the risk of multiple birth if many follicles are produced simultaneously. If this occurs, the insemination may need to be abandoned for that cycle, and treatment recommenced in a following month. To avoid this risk of multiple birth most units monitor FSH injections with regular ultrasound, usually four to six visits before insemination. It is therefore quite an invasive treatment.

Occasionally a split ejaculate will obtain richer sperm. Some men with a low sperm count may have a concentration of their most active sperm during the first part of the ejaculate. To produce a split ejaculate the man masturbates the first part of his ejaculate into one pot and then switches to a new pot for the rest. Not very easy in practice, but it can give improved sperm samples.

IUI may be used for a wide variety of reasons:

- The man has a marginally low sperm count or has sperm antibodies. AI has a limited place here, but it is worth trying before IVF. IVF is much more involved and expensive but gives evidence that the sperm are capable of fertilisation. If a treatment with IVF fails – but fertilisation occurred easily – it may be worth persisting with AI.
- When both partners have been tested and no significant abnormality has been found. This is a justified way of avoiding IVF and is a good initial option – particularly if ovulation is gently stimulated in each cycle. There is little value in IUI in these circumstances without

ovarian stimulation. For typical success rates see Chapter 6. Results are much less successful in older women – say, over 38 – who may be better to try IVF earlier because of their diminishing fertility.

- There may be problems with intercourse – or having sex at the fertile time. However, allowing sexual difficulties to persist in any partnership is fraught with frustration and risk for one or other partner. Therefore every attempt to get psychosexual or other help may be recommended. AI may be justified (with frozen sperm) if the male partner is away from home. This is not ideal, as it may cause considerable stress for the woman. Moreover, frozen sperm is never as fertile.

- When a man is able to have normal intercourse but has retrograde ejaculation. In this condition the sperm are not ejaculated from the end of the penis but into the bladder. In such circumstances, a drug can be taken by mouth to make the urine alkaline so that the sperm will survive. After orgasm, urine is collected, the sperm are filtered, washed and used for AI.

- When both partners both have a minor problem – for example, irregular ovulation, inability to have intercourse regularly or a slightly marginal sperm count.

- When the woman has severe upper vaginal or cervical scarring. The most common indication is possibly after a cone biopsy of the cervix when cancer cells are removed. IUI may also be tried if the cervix is unable to produce normal mucus giving a satisfactory environment in which the sperm would normally swim.

- In some cases where the woman does not ovulate regularly, but ovulates in response to drugs like clomiphene or FSH injections. When treatment with these drugs alone has failed – perhaps after four to six months – IUI may be added.

- For donor insemination. IUI is the better option for routine donor insemination. If there has been no success after nine cycles however, IVF with donor sperm may be appropriate, particularly for older women.

Although insemination causes little physical discomfort, there may be emotional pain. The process is clinical, unspontaneous and for some, humiliating. The man may find it hard to masturbate to order, and collecting a split ejaculate is difficult. The treatment may be embarrassing, with feelings of guilt, frustration and anger. A great deal of patience and understanding may be needed by both partners.

All insemination requires timing of ovulation. Temperature charting is inadequate. A good clinic will do blood tests or ultrasound, or both. To maximise the chances of the sperm being in the right place at the right time, insemination may be repeated two or three times each month. Most couples take several months to conceive by AI. A few find it so disruptive that they give up after a few months. In general if insemination has not worked after six attempts it is appropriate to try IVF.

Donor insemination (DI)

Donor insemination (DI) may be considered when a man is not producing any viable sperm. Most responsible doctors will not use DI unless there is no chance of pregnancy by other methods. It may also be suggested if the man carries a genetic disease as sperm from a donor free from the genetic abnormality can allow a couple to have unaffected children.

DI is not as successful as might be thought. Donated sperm has to be frozen for a six month quarantine period while tests are done to ensure the donor is free of serious illnesses. The freezing/thawing process undoubtedly reduces the fertility of the sperm, and few clinics achieve better than a five–twelve per cent chance of a pregnancy each month with donor sperm (see page 105). Many healthy, perfectly fertile women repeatedly fail to conceive with multiple insemination attempts.

The sperm donor

Sperm donors in Britain have traditionally been university students (mostly studying medicine) because access to them is easy. Roughly 75 per cent of British donors are students, and 25 per cent are married men with children. They are screened as carefully as possible for serious illness and infection. The height, build, hair colour, complexion and eyes of donors are recorded. Attempts are usually made to match the physical characteristics of the woman's partner, as well as his ethnic group and religion if requested. Most centres ensure that the blood group of the donor is also matched to avoid risks of the baby developing Rhesus disease.

Less attention is paid to what is just as important. University students, often achievers in a particular academic field, may not provide the most suitable match for the backgrounds of recipients. This kind of considera-tion is not often discussed by clinics undertaking this work.

Sperm donors are not always of proved fertility. Most have not had children, are unmarried and are probably not ready for a long-term relationship. Nor is there a way of establishing through screening that a particular donor is free of all genes for serious inherited diseases. It is now possible to screen them for cystic fibrosis and The Human Fertilisation and Embryology Authority has recommended that this should be part of all screening now. This is not always done and in any case, there are rare DNA variations of the cystic fibrosis defect for which there is no screening test possible. There is normally a genetic history of the donor's family available, but this does not guarantee freedom from a particular genetic trait.

Another serious concern about using students as donors is that they may possibly be promiscuous and at risk of contracting sexually trans-mitted infections. Even though sperm may be held in quarantine and donors are checked routinely for HIV and hepatitis, there is a remote possibility that they might contract an infection from a casual partner after they have been checked. This may occasionally happen and I have encountered a few female patients who seem to have contracted pelvic inflammatory disease during DI. In each case, an initial laparoscopy before DI showed completely normal tubes and ovaries, so their sub-sequent damage was possibly a result of exposure to infected semen. Fortunately, in recent years, clinics have improved the recruitment of donors. There is better screening and casual infection is rare.

If repeated inseminations with a particular donor's semen fail to produce a pregnancy, most clinics switch to a different donor. Donor programmes are likely to have a limited number of good fertile donors and inevitably clinics may repeatedly use semen from a donor of proved fertility. The fear that siblings conceived by DI might marry, unaware of their relationship to each other, resulted in a ruling that no donor should have his semen used more than ten times. The risk of consanguinity is remote, but exists as a faint possibility. For a discussion of the issues surrounding sperm donation, see page 147. Clinics offering donor insem-ination and national results are listed on page 232.

Egg donation

Total inability to produce eggs is not that rare. For example, a surprising number of young women – several thousand in the UK – suffer a pre-mature menopause. The ovary does not make follicles and therefore does not produce the female hormone oestrogen. Therefore these women, as well as being sterile, generally need hormone replacement therapy. This condition – which is mostly of unknown cause – can strike as early as the age of twenty and is distressing. Many afflicted young women feel as if they are not properly female.

Until IVF, there was no treatment for young menopausal women. Egg donation, which was first successfully done by Alan Trounson's group in 1984 in Monash University, Melbourne, Australia, proved revolutionary. Not only was it possible for these women to carry a baby, but treatment was surprisingly successful.

A key problem has been difficulty in finding egg donors. Egg donors have to go through the IVF process, at least in so far as having their ovaries stimulated and undergoing egg collection. This is a discouragement – no matter how altruistic the donor. Once the eggs are obtained, they are fertilised with the sperm of the recipient's partner and any resulting embryos are transferred to her uterus. Because most women who cannot produce eggs are not producing enough oestrogen, they usually are given hormones to stimulate the uterine lining sufficiently to enable an embryo to implant. Once the recipient becomes pregnant, the developing pregnancy will itself provide sufficient hormones to ensure its safe development.

Unlike donor insemination, egg donation involves both partners in any resulting pregnancy because the husband is providing half the genetic material. Though the infertile woman is not the genetic mother of her child, she carries it within her own body and gives birth to it.

Indications for egg donation

Egg donation is chiefly used for women whose own ovaries are not producing eggs. Apart from women entering an early menopause, other situations in which egg donation may be appropriate are:

- The woman's own eggs have repeatedly failed to fertilise during IVF. The presumption is that her eggs have an inherent abnormality preventing fertilisation.
- The woman's ovaries respond very badly to ovarian stimulation during IVF treatment or eggs cannot be collected because of scar tissue or ovarian cysts.
- The woman has no ovarian tissue, for example Turner's syndrome, the congenital disease caused by a woman having only one X chromosome (see page 93).
- Serious genetic disease in the recipient's family. If no gene probe exists to detect the defect, egg donation may offer the only means of having healthy children.
- Radiation during cancer treatment which has killed all the eggs in the ovaries. In a tiny percentage of women the ovaries may recover after irradiation; most, however, are made menopausal.

Procedure

Many women who need donor eggs may not be having periods, unless they are on hormone replacement therapy. This means that their endometrium, the uterine lining, is very thin. Even if an embryo was transferred, implantation might not take place. Therefore, for egg donation to work, it may be necessary to stimulate the uterus with hormones. Oestrogen and progesterone may therefore be given to the woman in a cyclical fashion, creating an artificial menstrual cycle. Donor eggs are then fertilised with the partner's sperm and embryos are transferred to the recipient's artificially stimulated uterus. It is usual practice to replace two embryos unless a patient has previously failed this treatment. Most donors, because they often produce more than two viable eggs, may supply eggs for two recipients simultaneously.

Success rate

Egg donation cycles are more likely to be successful than routine IVF treatments. A single IVF cycle, using a woman's own eggs, has on average only about a fourteen or fifteen per cent chance of resulting in the birth of a live baby. But if donor eggs are used, the success rates can be often doubled or tripled.

Egg donors are young women, under the age of thirty-five. As a woman ages, more of her eggs seem to develop genetic defects when they mature. Eggs from younger women fertilise more readily and produce embryos which are much more likely to implant. Miscarriage and defects such as Down's syndrome are slightly less common after egg donation.

One reason why egg donation is so successful may be because recipients are not exposed to the drugs used to stimulate the ovaries. In a routine IVF cycle it is possible that these drugs may have adverse effects on the uterus and its lining. Vigorous ovarian stimulation results in a large number of follicles being matured, but it also stimulates the ovaries to produce huge amounts of oestrogen. During a typical IVF cycle, the ovaries may produce five to ten times the normal amount of oestrogen. This gets into the bloodstream and is carried to the uterus, where it could result in the uterine lining becoming too thick and less able to allow the embryo to implant. In an egg donation cycle, the recipient of the fertilised eggs is not exposed to excess oestrogen, but is given precisely the right amount of this hormone to encourage the best uterine development.

It is of interest that recipients who are totally menopausal and not menstruating at all, may have a better chance of success of pregnancy with egg donation than menstruating women. Egg donation for menstruating recipients may possibly be more difficult because control and timing of endometrial development is harder.

Egg donors

There are many women who are seeking donated eggs, but a great shortage of egg donors. Very few women are prepared to be donors which is hardly surprising given the amount of commitment they need. Apart from the psychological and social issues, these factors include:

- Before going into a donor programme, egg donors will need to have a number of blood tests and possibly genetic screening to make certain that they are healthy. They will certainly have to be screened for viral infections such as hepatitis or HIV. This is an invasion of their privacy and naturally enough often causes misgivings.
- An egg donor has to undergo considerable medical treatment. She will need to take the drugs which are usually given to women during an IVF cycle, to make her ovaries produce as many eggs as possible. These drugs have side-effects which an infertile woman will tolerate because she knows that taking them will give her the only chance of a pregnancy. But it is entirely different for an altruistic donor. Fertility drugs can often make women unwell or depressed. Abdominal bloating and tenderness are common. Hot flushes and headaches are quite frequent. Very often taking the drugs disrupts the menstrual cycle, causing irregular bleeding for several months after treatment has stopped.
- During treatment with the drugs, the egg donor will need to have very careful, regular supervision. Even with it, fertility drugs can cause hyperstimulation (see page 216). She will need daily ultrasound assessment, and in addition, many hospitals also prefer recipients of fertility drugs to have repeated blood samples. Regular attendance at a hospital for all this is daunting, especially for a woman who may be bringing up a young family.
- Moreover, donors need an operation to remove the eggs from their ovaries. It may be relatively minor but it can result in post-operative pain. In addition, as with any anaesthetic procedure, there is always the slight risk of accidents such as bleeding.

Embryo donation

A number of frozen embryos, stored after successful IVF treatment, are preserved in liquid nitrogen banks. If the genetic parents have no further need for them, these embryos can, with consent, be donated to infertile couples who have had no success with their IVF treatment. Embryo donation has been described as a form of 'adoption in utero', but it does mean that the recipient has a chance of giving birth to her 'adopted' child and nurturing it from its earliest days.

In practice, embryo donation has never been a particularly common treatment, because most parents with spare embryos from an earlier IVF cycle have not wished to commit themselves to an act of donation. They have, naturally enough, wished to ensure that their own child-bearing is completed first. Embryos, in theory, should be capable of being frozen for several hundred years in liquid nitrogen, without damage. However, until recently, the law in Britain prevented the storage of embryos for longer than five years, and therefore, in practice, most embryos which might be used for another couple's treatment have been destroyed at the conclusion of the time limit. Although, with specific consent, this period can be extended now for a further five years, few donor embryos have been available for potential recipients. There are no statutory requirements in the USA.

Embryo donation is technically quite similar to egg donation. It involves careful cycle timing and the uterine lining may need priming with drugs beforehand to give the best chance of implantation.

Surrogacy

Some women have had their womb removed (hysterectomy) because of disease. Others may have a severely damaged uterus, perhaps because of previous infection of the lining of the womb into which a developing embryo implants. Severe uterine scarring may occur rarely after operations for benign tumours such as fibroids, and such women may be unlikely to carry a pregnancy successfully. On rare occasions a girl may be born with a congenitally deformed uterus which is so abnormal that later pregnancy is very unlikely. In these cases of severe uterine damage or malformation routine IVF is generally futile, and the only solution for such patients may be for another woman, possibly a friend or relative, to bear their baby.

Requests for surrogacy are very rare. Because they are so fraught with risk for all parties concerned, a great deal of careful advice, assessment and counselling is needed. There are also considerable dangers, not least of a tug-of-war between the surrogate mother and the parents concerned. The feelings of children born in this situation have never, to my knowledge, been analysed.

There are two kinds of surrogacy. The surrogate mother's own eggs may be fertilised naturally after artificial insemination from the adopting male partner. In its most primitive form, this kind of approach does not of course require any medical supervision. It is unknown how often couples may enter into this kind of arrangement in Britain – but it is clear that it is not that uncommon. A difficulty will, of course, occur when the child is born. He or she will have to be adopted by the commissioning parents, and what was a very private arrangement will be forced into the open.

Many women with a damaged uterus, or even those born with no uterus at all, have normal ovaries which produce perfectly good eggs. When IVF is used, an egg taken from the ovary of a woman with a damaged or absent uterus may be fertilised *in vitro* in the usual way. Such a woman requires the full monitoring associated with IVF. The surrogate will also need careful surveillance until the time is right for transfer into her uterus. The procedure is made tricky because, in order to use fresh rather than frozen embryos, the cycles of the two women need synchronisation. Once an embryo has been produced, the surrogate undergoes transfer and carries the baby. At delivery she hands it over to the genetic parents for adoption. For a discussion of the problems concerned with surrogacy, see page 185.

Gamete intrafallopian transfer (GIFT)

This treatment involves stimulation of the ovaries to produce eggs, taking them from the ovaries and mixing them with sperm. Immediately after mixing they are placed in the fallopian tube of the woman. This is done before fertilisation. The treatment is different from IVF because the eggs are not fertilised, nor developed into embryos outside the body. Instead, fertilisation occurs in the natural environment, the fallopian tube. Although fertilisation in the natural fluids of the body may seem an advantage of GIFT, the results are generally worse than with IVF.

The treatment, unlike IVF, does not bypass the fallopian tube and consequently is not truly appropriate in cases of tubal disease. GIFT is most effective when more than one egg has been collected and mixed with the sperm. Therefore, as with IVF, there is a risk of overstimulation of the ovaries. It also needs an operation to collect the eggs. These are usually collected by laparoscopy (see page 37), rather than ultrasound, because the surgeon needs to use the laparoscope to put the eggs and sperm into the fallopian tube.

The main reason given for GIFT treatment is usually in cases of un-explained infertility. As it bypasses the cervix, it may also be used when there is a problem with the cervical mucus. But it is not nearly as good a treatment as IVF, although it is just as demanding and expensive. It is obviously better to transfer embryos knowing that fertilisation and embryo development are normal, rather than unfertilised eggs which may or may not develop. In my view most GIFT attempts are something of a waste of resources because IVF gives better information. It generally has more chance of success in infertility units which have access to IVF equipment. It has to be regretted that a number of National Health Service units in Britain are providing GIFT, and thus offering expensive second-class treatment simply because they don't have IVF facilities. However, as access to IVF has improved in recent years, GIFT has become less fashionable. Because the procedure does not produce an embryo inside the body, it can be done in any hospital and is not licensed by law. Oddly, the Human Fertilisation and Embryology Authority (HFEA) has no control over it. It may also have an advantage for some patients – for example, religious Catholics – because, as embryos are not produced *in vitro*, it is more acceptable to the Church. However, this is still procreation without sexual intercourse which may present religious problems for some couples.

Zygote intrafallopian transfer (ZIFT)

This is a variation on GIFT treatment where the unfertilised egg, mixed with the sperm, is placed in the fallopian tube. A zygote is a fertilised egg. In zygote fallopian transfer (ZIFT), eggs are collected as for IVF, fertilised outside the body *in vitro*, and as soon as they are fertilised, one or two, or possibly three, are selected for transfer into the fallopian tube. This normally requires using a laparoscopy.

The thinking behind ZIFT is that by placing the very early fertilised egg into the fallopian tube, it will be in its most natural environment, rather than in a culture dish in an oven. People who advocate ZIFT also feel that the certainty that fertilisation has occurred overcomes a major hurdle associated with, say, GIFT.

In practice however there seems little advantage in ZIFT. It is as complicated as IVF, and like GIFT requires a laparoscopic operation. Although the early statistics were promising, there is little evidence to suggest that the overall chance of a pregnancy is any better with ZIFT than with any other assisted reproductive treatment. Moreover, if there is any damage to the fallopian tube at all, or any possible disease of the fallopian tube causing the infertility, there is a serious risk of ectopic pregnancy.

Transuterine fallopian transfer (TUFT) and synchronised hysteroscopic intrafallopian transfer (SHIFT)

A variation of ZIFT is TUFT or SHIFT. TUFT stands for 'transuterine fallopian transfer' and SHIFT for 'synchronised hysteroscopic intra-fallopian transfer'. In these variations, a laparoscopy is avoided. Once the operation to collect the eggs has been completed, the eggs are fertilised outside the body and then immediately transferred into the fallopian tube through the uterus from below. A variation of this technique uses a hysteroscope – a telescope inserted into the uterine cavity – hence the name SHIFT. Once again, as is so often commonly the case with these technologies, early results and claims for success were encouraging, but as more patients were treated the reported success rates fell substantially. There seems little to commend them, and I think that very few units still use these techniques.

Tubal insemination

As far as I am aware, tubal insemination was first performed at The Hammersmith Hospital in 1970, many years before IVF had been invented. The late Professor McClure Brown used to ask us, as his trainee assistants, to prepare certain infertile patients by stimulating ovulation using clomiphene. Just before ovulation, the husband's sperm was collected and then a laparoscopic examination was scheduled in the operating theatre. I well remember many lengthy and painstaking attempts to use the laparoscope to direct a fine piece of plastic tubing containing the sperm, into the fallopian tube. Professor Brown's idea was that by placing the sperm in the tube, it would be closest to the egg at the time of ovulation. As far as I know, he never published this work, but there were occasional pregnancies. Looking back at these historical trials, I now recognise that the patients on whom we tried these techniques were usually quite unsuitable and that may have been why the success rate was so low. Most of them had tubal problems, and many others had quite poor sperm quality.

In the mid-1980s, the technique was reinvented by a number of clinicians and called 'direct intraperitoneal insemination', or 'tubal insem-ination'. However, in most cases the attempts to do this were rather crude

– the sperm was mostly just injected into the abdomen – and I do not think that many of these patients had much chance of a pregnancy. Once *in vitro* fertilisation became more successful, intraperitoneal and tubal insemination were discontinued.

Tubal insemination could still have some merit and might be worth re-exploring. It avoids many of the complexities of IVF and the insemination could now be done by fine tubing through the cervix and uterus, and into the entrance of the tube from below. However, as far as I am aware, there has been little or no recent experience with this treatment.

Alternatives not involving assisted reproduction

Encouraging ovulation

Where the cause of infertility is a failure to ovulate, the specialist may recommend a course of drugs (see below). Except in women with an early menopause, this treatment induces ovulation in about 80 per cent of women. However, although ovulation may be established, not everybody gets a successful pregnancy. Around 65 per cent of couples with these treatments actually succeed.

Clomiphene

This is the standard 'fertility pill'. It is usually marketed as Clomid or Serophene. It has some properties similar to oestrogen and was developed in an attempt to find a contraceptive pill that did not have the oestrogen-like side-effects associated with oestrogens. However, in early trials some rats who had been given the drug got pregnant rather easily and so its future as a contraceptive was clearly over. Subsequently it was noticed that the rats who had been given it had become, on average, more fertile and therefore further tests were done. Finally, in 1961, Dr Greenblatt and colleagues in the USA, established the value of clomiphene for women who fail to ovulate.

Clomiphene is a good first-time treatment. It is cheap and free from major side-effects. It rarely causes multiple births because it is only a weak stimulant. It promotes ovulation by stimulating natural release of FSH from the pituitary. This makes the ovaries work harder to produce follicles. But because clomiphene is an anti-oestrogen, it can thicken cervical mucus, making the cervix unresponsive to sperm. It can also interfere with the growth of the uterine lining, and possibly prevent the embryo from implanting. Also, overstimulation with clomiphene can occasionally make the ovaries cystic. For these reasons, its use requires supervision.

One concern with clomiphene is possibly a slight risk of ovarian cancer (see also page 19). Three years ago, an article in *The New England Journal of Medicine*, a much respected journal in the United States, suggested that women who had taken clomiphene for a very long time might have a slightly higher risk of ovarian cancer than average. There was certainly no definite evidence of this, unless a woman had been taking it continuously for more than one year. Nor was there evidence that this drug was associated with any other cancers, including the womb or the breast.

It is rather difficult to know what to make of this report, as there have been no others confirming its conclusions. The number of patients followed up was not particularly large and the risks still remained very small. It must be remembered that infertile women, who have either not been fertile or have not had children, are known to be at slightly higher risk of ovarian cancers in any case. Consequently, analysis of the risk is difficult and responsible medical opinion is strongly of the view that clomiphene, given under supervision and for less than one year, is a completely safe drug.

Usually one tablet (50 mg) is taken every day for five days, starting from the first or second day of menstruation. If the cycle is much longer than 28 days, clomiphene may be given from the fifth day for five days. The dose may be increased (two tablets daily) if there is no positive response.

There are several symptoms which may indicate ovulation: breast tenderness, mid-cycle discomfort in the abdomen, vaginal discharge near ovulation time, painful and more regular periods. But none of these are conclusive proof that ovulation has taken place, so tests to check that ovulation really is occurring should be done. The best method is ultrasound. Not only does it accurately confirm ovulation, but also it will detect any cysts. A blood progesterone test is often used, but is not reliable. Clomiphene can stimulate the production of more than one follicle simultaneously, without ovulation occurring. The combined amounts of progesterone that these follicles produce together may raise the blood progesterone to an ovulatory value (30nmols or more) even although an egg has not been shed.

A side-effect of clomiphene is hot flushes. Abdominal discomfort may occur around the time of ovulation. A few women get frequent or irregular periods, and if this happens they should generally stop taking the drug. Cysts which may develop will not be serious, but the drug should be stopped to give the ovary a chance to recover. Some people may just feel unwell while taking it. There are drugs similar to clomiphene which can be taken instead. These include tamoxifen (Tamofen) and cyclofenil (Rehibin). They may have fewer side-effects but they are more expensive.

Clomiphene should generally be discontinued if a pregnancy has not occurred within six to nine months. There is very little value indeed in taking it for longer than one year. In thirty years of experience, I can remember only a very few women becoming pregnant with this drug after longer periods of time. If it does not restore ovulation, it should be stopped sooner.

Gonadotrophins

Human menopausal gonadotrophin (HMG) and pure follicle stimulating hormone (FSH)

An important breakthrough in hormone research was the discovery in 1960 that during the menopause the pituitary pours out the hormones LH and FSH to stimulate the flagging ovaries. Human menopausal gonadotrophin (HMG), originally marketed as Pergonal or Humegon, was the first mixture of these hormones to be used, although it is FSH which is the active ingredient. Although effective, these drugs are so powerful they must be given under close supervision. Usually they are reserved for cases where clomiphene has failed. But for some women they may be used as an initial treatment, particularly for those not having periods.

HMG is derived biologically. That is to say, it is purified from the urine of women who are excreting high amounts of FSH. In practice, the main source has been the urine of women who are menopausal – mostly women living in convents or in similar communal organisations. There have been many problems with this kind of biological source. First of all, supply, usually from nunneries, has waxed and waned around Europe. Secondly, the FSH so obtained has been difficult to purify, even using the most sophisticated chemical techniques. Because the drug contains some foreign proteins, adverse side-effects, such as painful injection sites and skin rashes, have not been uncommon. Moreover, because the drug is biologically derived and is never absolutely pure, the strength tends to vary. One batch of HMG might be extremely effective, but another much less so – the same dose stimulating the ovary much less well.

For all these reasons, the major drug companies involved in marketing FSH in its various forms did a great deal of work to find a pure form of the drug. During the 1990s, two leading manufacturers, Serono and Organon, managed to set up a system using genetically engineered animal cells which produced pure FSH only. Pure genetically engineered FSH (or so-called recombinant FSH) has now virtually entirely replaced the earlier forms of the drugs. Initially great claims were made for these replacement drugs. They were said to be more powerful and effective. In practice, most clinicians believe that they are simply safer and less likely to have the side-effects associated with skin reactions and other reactions to foreign proteins. There is not much evidence that actual pregnancy rates have greatly increased with their use. Unfortunately, developing any new drug is very expensive and developing one that is genetically engineered is especially so. This new generation of drugs comes at a high price.

FSH is usually injected daily from the early part of the menstrual cycle until ovulation is imminent – usually about five to ten days later. When ovulation is just about to occur, a triggering injection of human chorionic gonadotrophin (HCG) is given. HCG is similar to LH, the hormone which initiates ovulation. Without this the ovary will not usually shed the egg.

During a course of FSH, it is usual to conduct regular ultrasound measurements of the ovarian follicles and often to measure the level of oestrogen in the blood as well. Without this close monitoring HMG or FSH can be dangerous. Some women get hyperstimulation syndrome (see page 17). There is also a serious risk of multiple ovulation with the complication of multiple birth, but by monitoring the response of the ovaries carefully, the triggering dose of HCG can be withheld if there are too many follicles.

Because FSH is a very expensive drug, and proper monitoring with ultrasound adds to its cost, most clinics offer the treatment for only three months at a time. The treatment then needs to be reviewed. A typical month's drug bill can be £300–£800. If conception does not follow after six cycles in which ovulation has occurred, treatment should be stopped. There is a less than ten per cent chance that continued treatment will be successful and under these circumstances IVF is usually indicated.

In a normally fertile woman the pituitary gland releases FSH and LH in pulses every 60–90 minutes. Although the significance of this is not understood, some doctors have suggested that treatment with FSH may be more effective if it mimics this natural process in which case the patient wears an electric pump attached to a syringe, which automatically delivers doses at appropriate intervals. Such 'pump therapy' might be helpful, particularly in cases of polycystic ovary disease, and for women who are producing very small amounts of FSH and LH of their own.

Releasing hormone (LHRH)

The production of LH and FSH from the pituitary gland is normally triggered by the secretion of releasing hormones in the hypothalamus – a small area at the base of the brain. This stimulus occurs in regular pulses and results in the pituitary gland releasing pulses of LH and FSH. The injection of LH-releasing hormone (LHRH) at regular intervals has been shown to be a particularly effective treatment in those rare cases where the communication between the hypothalamus and the pituitary gland is not working properly.

One advantage of LHRH therapy is that it is less likely to result in multiple pregnancy. It merely stimulates the pituitary gland, leaving the pituitary to release LH and FSH in the quantities naturally required. If it is indicated, there is every reason to continue this kind of treatment for at least six months to a year before considering IVF.

Buserelin, Lupron

Like LHRH, these drugs which are chemically similar, work by initially stimulating the pituitary gland to produce more FSH and LH. After several days of use they suppress the action of the pituitary. They are taken in the form of a nasal spray, which needs to be taken first thing in the morning and last thing at night and usually up to four hourly during the day.

Because Buserelin is basically a pituitary gland suppressant, it is not generally used on its own as a fertility treatment. Indeed, drugs like Buserelin, which stop the pituitary making its ovarian stimulating hormones, are used mainly to suppress the ovaries as well. It can be given to stop ovarian function so that conditions like endometriosis, or fibroids, regress. Both of these conditions are dependent for their growth on the presence of oestrogen, and once the ovaries are suppressed, endometriosis tends to disappear and fibroids to shrink. As soon as the drug is stopped this temporary menopause ceases. This is reassuring in one way, but it generally means the return of endometriosis and the regrowth of fibroids.

Buserelin is chiefly used in conjunction with drugs like FSH which stimulate the ovary. In some women, particularly those with polycystic ovaries, it may be more effective to give Buserelin initially to suppress pituitary function and then to follow this up with FSH. Then the ovary may become maximally responsive. This is the principle used in stimulation during IVF treatment, but it can be also used simply to induce ovulation in selected cases. The approach has many disadvantages. Firstly it may cause too much stimulation with too many eggs. For this reason it is more suitable for IVF than merely for the induction of ovulation. Secondly, all this family of drugs are expensive and require very extensive monitoring.

Progesterone

In some cases the woman's uterine lining (the endometrium) is too thin for an embryo to implant, perhaps because the ovary has not produced enough progesterone after ovulation. Some doctors try to make up for this deficiency by giving the patient extra progesterone in the form of an injection or vaginal pessary. Others give injections of HCG which encourages the ovaries to produce their own progesterone. But there is little evidence that these treatments work except on a very occasional basis.

Wedge resection and ovarian drilling

Occasionally when drug treatment fails, it is possible to stimulate ovulation by removing a piece of ovarian tissue. Quite why this works is unclear, but possibly it alters the production of growth factors in the ovary which in turn affect the development of the follicles. The advent of the laparoscope and microsurgery make it possible to perform this operation without the risk of adhesion formation, which can damage the tubes. One method which works well is to drill the ovarian capsule during a laparoscopy. The burning or drilling can be done with an electric needle or with a fine laser beam. There is no evidence that the method of drilling makes any difference to the success rate. If pregnancy has not occurred within one year of this treatment, IVF should certainly be considered.

Tubal microsurgery

The use of the microscope and fine instruments have revolutionised treatment of damage around the fallopian tubes and ovaries. Unfortunately, microsurgery requires particular specialist skill from the surgeon and too few doctors are trained in it and unskilled surgery in the wrong hands, is most likely to cause more damage, for example by causing adhesions. These factors, together with the increasing availability of IVF, has made microsurgery unfashionable. This is a very great pity indeed, because in the right patients, microsurgery is frequently far more effective than IVF. Moreover, it is a treatment for the infertility itself. Successful tubal microsurgery allows the successful patient to get pregnant after natural intercourse, and to become pregnant at regular intervals when needed. Moreover, there is no risk of multiple pregnancy or the other complications associated with IVF. It is deeply to be regretted that more doctors do not consider this treatment, or consider referring patients to a centre where this kind of treatment has a good success rate.

The main microsurgical procedures are:

- *Division or removal of tubal adhesions.* This operation is known as an *adhesiolysis* when it is used to remove adhesions in the ovaries or uterus, and as a *salpingolysis* when the fallopian tubes are involved. In good hands and with proper selection of patients, the chance of a successful pregnancy is between 40–60 per cent after this surgery
- *Opening the ovarian end of the tubes.* Blockage of the fallopian tubes usually involves the fimbria (the end of the tube, near the ovary). The fimbria pick up the egg from the ovary and pass it down the tube. When they are blocked, the tube swells up with fluid and can be badly damaged. The operation to open up the tube is known as a salpingostomy. If the tubes are heavily scarred or the tubal lining has been damaged, it is generally best to proceed straight to IVF. If, after proper selection of cases, salpingostomy is performed with microsurgery, up to 40 per cent of patients will conceive naturally and have a baby. Unfortunately, the chance of ectopic pregnancy is also increased to about six per cent of all pregnancies.
- *Blocked tubes near the uterus.* The fallopian tubes can become blocked where they join the uterus. This area is called the cornu (or horn). Until the advent of microsurgery the standard operation involved removing the cornu and crudely connecting the tube to the uterus. Less than twenty per cent of patients who had this operation conceived. In the modern operation, called cornual anastomosis, the blocked or damaged part of the tube is removed by microsurgery and the healthy remainder is stitched back together with stitches finer than a human hair. Between 45 and 65 per cent of the women who have the operation will go on to have a live baby. The chance of an ectopic pregnancy afterwards is only about three per cent. Consequently, this is a more successful treatment than IVF.
- *Reversal of sterilisation.* Women who have been sterilised can have their tubes reconstituted by microsurgery. The chance of a live birth

afterwards is between 65 and 95 per cent, depending mostly on how the original sterilisation was done. Unless there are very good reasons to the contrary, microsurgery should always be tried in such cases before IVF, but like all microsurgery it is crucial that it is done by a surgeon who does this kind of surgery regularly. It is both cheaper and more effective than IVF and allows repeated pregnancy.

Undergoing tubal microsurgery

The standard procedure for tubal microsurgery is to make a cut across the pubic-hair line – a 'bikini' incision – which after six months leaves only a very faint scar. Microsurgery is performed with such precision that most patients recover far more quickly than after conventional operations. The hospital stay is about three or four days. There is some pain, although it is not severe. The worst discomfort is usually in the first two days caused by the swelling of the abdomen with wind, and this is easy to deal with.

After seven days, the stitches can be removed. This takes a few seconds and is painless. It can take four or five weeks to recover completely, although some people feel back to normal after only a couple of weeks. There is no harm in having sex as soon as both partners feel up to it, but for the first two weeks after leaving hospital it is best not to place too much strain on the abdomen by heavy lifting or vigorous exercise. Although the tubes themselves cannot be damaged, over-exertion will delay the healing of the wound and make the abdomen sore. The amount of discomfort and inconvenience after microsurgery is no more, and often less, than that with IVF.

Regular attendance at the clinic after the operation is essential. At The Hammersmith Hospital we like to see our patients every three months until they get pregnant or decide to try alternative treatments. This enables us to maximise fertility by keeping an eye on ovulation and sperm counts.

If there are any gynaecological symptoms after surgery such as pain or irregular bleeding, a doctor – preferably the specialist – should be consulted as soon as possible, since any inflammation or infection needs to be treated at once. As soon as a woman thinks she is pregnant, she should let her specialist know. As we have seen, tubal surgery, like IVF, slightly increases the chance of ectopic pregnancy, and it may be wise to monitor the early stages of the pregnancy through ultrasound for this reason.

Women who do not get pregnant immediately after tubal surgery always worry about how soon to try IVF. This, I think, depends on a number of factors, the most important of which will be how well the surgeon feels the surgery has gone. A second consideration is the age of the woman. In the case of younger women (under 36) we would certainly recommend trying by natural means for at least a year after surgery. Some of our patients have conceived two or three years after surgery, and after that have had regular pregnancies. We have had one patient who did not conceive for eighteen months after surgery, and then had six pregnancies with a live baby in each case each year following.

In some cases, it may be worth assessing the state of the fallopian tubes by laparoscopy six months to one year after the surgery to make certain they are still open and that there are not too many adhesions. In a woman over 36 it may well be worthwhile considering a laparoscopy earlier than this.

Women who have had tubal surgery must understand that often it is not an instant solution. It is very easy to feel dispirited at the start of a period especially if it is a day or two late. And it is probably as well to remember that following any fertility surgery the chance of conception each month is never much higher than ten per cent, compared to the normal chance of fifteen–eighteen per cent in women who never had any tubal damage or scar tissue in the pelvis.

One of the problems in nearly all women who have had tubal damage of any kind, particularly if there has been inflammation, is that their ovaries will have also been damaged. For this reason, it is now recognised that many women who have considerable tubal damage, even after correction following microsurgery will have a slightly reduced chance of achieving a pregnancy. IVF after any tubal disease is also slightly less likely to be successful.

Laparoscopic surgery

This alternative to open microsurgery is becoming increasingly common. The laparoscope is introduced through a small hole in the navel, and the fine surgical instruments through small holes made just above the pubic-hair line. Long scissors, or an electrical current or a laser are used to cut any adhesions. A fine jet of fluid is used to wash away any blood, which is then sucked out by a small tube. Bleeding is controlled using a diathermy machine or a laser. It is a particularly useful way of dealing with endometriosis or cysts in the ovaries.

The advantage of laparoscopic surgery over microsurgery is the speed with which patients recover. There is no abdominal wound requiring time to heal and therefore generally only an overnight stay in hospital is necessary.

Laparoscopic surgery is most successful when there are adhesions in the pelvis. It is less satisfactory for opening the fallopian tube at its outer end, and impossible for opening the inner end of the fallopian tube. We have found that although the recovery after laparoscopic surgery is rather quicker than it is with the open microsurgical approach, the success rate is lower. At The Hammersmith Hospital, laparoscopic surgery has resulted in approximately 30 per cent of patients becoming pregnant after removal of adhesions and it is much less successful after salpingostomy.

Tubal catheterisation

Tubal catheterisation is sometimes used for those patients who have their tubes blocked near the uterine end, the cornu, where it enters the uterus. The procedure involves passing a fine wire probe or dilator into the tube from below using X-ray equipment. Very optimistic results have been quoted for this procedure, but in our hands at The Hammersmith Hospital, we have been unconvinced of its value. Its main advantage would seem to be that it is an out-patient procedure. Dilating the blocked part of the tube alone is certainly not going to remove any diseased tissue, so on theoretical grounds such an approach will not seem to be particularly valuable. Advocates of the operation claim that perhaps 40 per cent of their patients conceive successfully.

Treating endometriosis

Endometriosis is a condition where the lining of the uterus, the endometrium, grows not only in the uterus but also in the abdomen. Occasionally, it can lead to adhesions or severe scarring of the tubes. Mild or moderate endometriosis only needs to be treated when the woman is suffering pain or where there is bad scarring or distortion of the tissues around the tubes and ovaries.

Spots of endometriosis can be burned with diathermy (heat generated by a high frequency electric current) or a laser during laparoscopy at the same time as a diagnosis is made. This approach can be a means of treating endometriosis which is causing cysts on the ovary. In expert hands between 40–70 per cent of women will conceive after laparoscopic surgery for endometriosis.

Endometriosis can also be treated with drugs. The endometrium normally grows under the influence of oestrogen. Drugs such as Buserelin which suppress ovarian activity cause the endometriosis to melt away. The advantage of drug therapy is that it may avoid the need for surgery, but drugs can have unpleasant side-effects. Also, conception is virtually impossible while they are being taken and endometriosis is likely to grow again once the treatment has been stopped for more than a few months.

In general, when the endometriosis is mild, IVF has a very good rate of success. At our clinic, treatment of endometriosis by IVF has consistently been about five per cent more successful than all other IVF treatments except those treatments involving male infertility. If the endometriosis is very mild, surgery probably will not be of benefit and IVF will become the treatment of choice. When the endometriosis is more pronounced, IVF is not so successful and surgery may be worth considering first. One problem with IVF is that the hormonal stimulation of the ovaries used to get large numbers of eggs may also cause the endometriosis to grow more vigorously. It is not uncommon, therefore, for women with endometriosis to have more pain after a failed IVF treatment cycle. They may also have more irregular menstrual cycles. One paradox is that any treatment, including IVF, which results in pregnancy will help the endometriosis to get better. This is because during pregnancy the pregnancy hormones suppress the growth of endometrial tissue including pockets of endometriosis implanted outside the womb.

Treating uterine problems

Fibroids

Fibroids can cause infertility particularly if they distort the uterine cavity, displace the ovaries or block the uterine end of the fallopian tubes. They are best removed by a microsurgical operation called a myomectomy. The fibroids are carefully dissected away from the uterine muscle and the space left and the muscle of the uterus is meticulously repaired with stitches. The uterus may bleed and extra blood is usually on hand as a safety precaution, but a transfusion is very rarely needed. When a microsurgical approach is used, and the surgeon has specially designed instruments, the risk of any blood loss at all is really minimal. There is no question that myomectomy is best done by a fully trained, specially qualified, fertility expert. Under these circumstances, the operation is much more likely to be successful, there is much less likelihood of scar tissue, and there will be more chance of a pregnancy afterwards. When this operation is performed on women under the age of 38, about 65 per cent conceive afterwards, but it is far less successful after this age, with only about 35 per cent becoming pregnant.

Some surgeons advocate myomectomy using the laparoscope. Using laparoscopic instruments or a laser, the fibroids are shelled out or burnt away. This may cause less post-operative discomfort but laparoscopic myomectomy can cause serious damage. Many women treated by laparoscopic myomectomy at other centres have come to The Hammersmith Hospital. They frequently have severe adhesions in the abdomen and the uterine healing is often rather poor. Not surprisingly, our impression is that far fewer of these women become pregnant than those having open surgery. It is also true that a laparoscopic myomectomy takes longer, and is rather more dangerous.

It is surprising how many women are offered IVF when they have fibroids in their uterus. Obviously, a small fibroid which is not distorting the uterine cavity is insignificant and unlikely to make any difference. But it does not make any sense to have complex and expensive IVF if the uterus is distorted by fibroids. Under these circumstances, it is preferable to correct the uterine deformity first. After all, the embryo has to implant and grow in the uterus and if the uterus is abnormal this is less likely to happen.

Congenital abnormalities

These conditions may often require surgery. The human uterus grows from two tubes fusing together. Most congenital abnormalities are the result of incomplete fusion. They can cause infertility and miscarriage as well. On rare occasions an open operation called utriculoplasty may be needed. About 65 per cent of women will go on to become pregnant after such an operation. Most cases of abnormality are not that severe and can be tackled from below by day-case surgery. The most common abnormality is a septate uterus. In this condition, the upper part of the uterine cavity is deformed by a septum – a division in the centre of the uterus. This can usually be cut with the aid of a hysteroscope passed into the uterus from the vagina. There may be some vaginal bleeding, but probably no more than during a period. Recuperation after the operation is swift. Only if the septum is very large will the surgeon elect to remove it by opening the uterus from above, after opening up the abdomen. The chance of pregnancy afterwards is about 75 per cent.

There is no question that IVF should not be tried until reasonable attempts have been made to correct any uterine abnormalities. This advice includes treatment of those which are congenital. The success rates of surgery are so good in these cases that IVF is simply unjustified. One of the commonest reasons for IVF failing is, in our experience, an undiagnosed congenital deformity of the uterus which was missed, because no X-ray (hysterosalpingogram) of the uterus was done before IVF was commenced. I feel like weeping when I see a woman who has had four or five failed attempts at IVF only to find that a simple day-case procedure to correct uterine problems was all that was needed in the first place.

Internal adhesions (synechiae or Asherman's syndrome)

Internal adhesions often cause the wall of the uterine cavity to stick together. They are best diagnosed by hysterosalpingogram (HSG). They can usually be separated with the aid of a hysteroscope and special scissors or a laser. The operation can be done as a day-case under anaesthesia. It may need to be repeated, sometimes more than once, and it may be necessary to insert a plastic coil into the uterus for a few weeks to keep the uterine walls apart. The chances of pregnancy afterwards is about 70 per cent. IVF is never indicated in patients with these kinds of adhesions until every reasonable attempt at correcting them has been made.

Polyps

These are fleshy, grape-like growths on the wall of the inside of the uterus. They are not very common and can be removed by a D & C (dilation of the cervix and curettage), or 'scrape', on the rare occasions when they are a cause of infertility.

Adenomyosis

With this condition the uterus becomes scarred when its muscle is invaded by lining tissue (the endometrium). Surgery is usually ineffective as the tissue cannot normally be removed without damaging the uterus. As in the case of endometriosis, drugs which suppress ovarian activity will cause the tissue to melt away, but of course will at the same time hinder pregnancy. Women with this condition have about a 35 per cent chance of getting pregnant at best. Sadly IVF has a poor chance of success with this condition; depending on its severity success rates in our unit vary from five to fifteen per cent.

4
Male fertility treatments involving IVF

It is said that *in vitro* fertilisation has been the single biggest advance in the treatment of infertility this century. That is undoubtedly true, but perhaps the biggest impact of IVF has been in the treatment of male infertility. It is remarkable to consider that until only a few years ago, most forms of male infertility were virtually untreatable. When on rare occasions evidence-based treatment was possible, the results were often entirely haphazard. IVF has changed that, because it allows direct access to the egg, manipulation of the sperm and the egg together, and visual assessment of fertilisation. For the first time, it has been possible to conduct a treatment knowing that fertilisation has occurred, and that a fertilised egg is in the uterus.

In the early days of IVF, fertilisation was capable of being somewhat enhanced, by placing a single egg in a droplet which contained more sperm than would normally surround the egg in its natural environment, the fallopian tube. It soon became obvious that it was often possible to achieve fertilisation in an artificial environment when men had relatively low sperm counts. The greatest development though, came with the ability to inject a sperm directly into the egg. Intracytoplasmic sperm injection has completely changed understanding of the treatment of male infertility. From being the least successful of all fertility treatments, the treatment of male infertility is now widely regarded as one of the most promising. Indeed, the recent improvement in the overall success rate of IVF has been largely because of improvements in the treatment of infertile males.

Intracytoplasmic sperm injection (ICSI)

Early work in this field started in the 1980s in animal eggs. Researchers succeeded in fertilising mice eggs by injecting single sperm into them. A sperm was sucked up into a fine glass needle, which was passed through the outer coat of the egg (the zona pellucida) and then directly into the substance of the egg (the cytoplasm). But this method was initially considered too dangerous to be used for humans. It was feared that there might be genetic damage to the egg, or that an abnormal sperm which had not been filtered out by natural protective processes might be injected.

Then, in the late 1980s, Dr Simon Fishel, at Nottingham University, developed a technique in humans which involved injecting sperm just under the egg's outer shell (zona). From here it might penetrate the cytoplasm on its own. His argument was based on the observation that many sperm of impaired motility still had sufficient movement to enter the egg, provided that the hard outer shell had first been penetrated. He felt that this means of fertilisation would be safer than direct injection. There would be no disruption of the egg itself, and there would still be some degree of selection of sperm, as the very damaged sperm would be unlikely to be able to penetrate the cytoplasm.

The refusal of the authorities in Britain to license a pilot scheme on humans forced him to pioneer his technique of sub-zonal sperm injection (SUZI) in Italy. Soon a number of once despairing couples were giving birth to completely normal babies. But SUZI would eventually be superseded by intracytoplasmic sperm injection (ICSI), the method which had originally been pioneered earlier in mice. ICSI completely replaced SUZI because it became rapidly obvious that it was very much more successful. It also had the advantage of needing only a single sperm for each egg to be injected. Early fears of the risk of genetic damage were assuaged when the first children were born. The group who were mostly responsible for the successful development of ICSI were the scientists at The Free University of Brussels, in Belgium, in a team lead by Professor André van Steirteghem.

ICSI is without question the greatest advance to have been made in helping the treatment of infertile males. Even if a man can produce only a single sperm, then ICSI may theoretically be able to help. His sperm do not even need to be able to move or to be fully mature. Couples whose only previous chance of having a baby was through DI can now take advantage of this treatment. Because the sperm do not need to be mature, even men who have a total blockage of the epididymis – the fine tube from the testes – or of any part of the male tubing from the testes – can be helped by sucking sperm directly from the blocked tubing or from the testicle itself.

The human egg is only 100 microns in diameter, thinner than a human hair and invisible to the naked eye. When it is first taken from the ovary, it is surrounded by two or three million sticky helper cells, which provide essential nutrients and remove waste products from the egg. All of these have to be removed under the microscope before sperm injection can begin. Once the egg has been cleaned, it has to be held rigidly under the microscope so that its outer zona can be penetrated.

ICSI requires exquisitely delicate manipulation with fine instruments. Two types of pipette are mainly needed. The fine holding pipette is about 0.04 millimetres across and gentle suction is applied to hold the egg immovable. The injection pipette is very much finer. Its internal diameter is hardly wider than the sperm head which is to be picked up, and it holds the sperm tail immobilised. Its tip is bevelled so it can penetrate the egg without disturbing its cytoplasm.

These glass pipettes are held rigidly in metal micromanipulators which isolate them from the operator's hands and allow very precise, controlled movements. Suction through the pipettes is done using syringes which are often mounted with the barrel of the syringe attached to a screw thread, to allow limited and precise suction. To avoid vibration – even someone walking in a corridor thirty metres away can disturb the procedure – most laboratories mount the microscope and micromanipulators on a specially isolated table which is cushioned from shocks in a variety of ways. Because equipment failure can occur most laboratories will have two such set-ups. As each workstation may cost around £50,000, this treatment is not cheap to establish.

Obviously, picking up a sperm in such a tiny fragile glass tube is excessively difficult, particularly when the sperm is capable of some movement. Even sperm which show limited viability will move around, so steps have to be taken to control their movement. Consequently, the sperm are immersed in a viscous fluid which prevents the sperm tail from thrashing around. The tail can then be crushed with the end of a pipette and once the sperm are immobilised in this way, it is relatively easy to suck them into the tip of the fine glass tube.

Injection is done by a sudden but controlled, thrusting movement. The sperm-holding pipette breaks through the zona of the egg, and then through the membrane surrounding the substance of the egg, the cyto-plasm. The nucleus of the egg must be left undamaged, and care must be taken not to go right through the egg to the other side. Injection of the sperm head must be gentle to minimise disturbance, and withdrawal of the needle after injection carefully controlled. It takes several minutes to inject each egg, and embryologists who are starting to learn the technique take longer. A patient who yields very many eggs may need well over an hour of bench time even when the laboratory is running smoothly. Treating more than one or two patients in a single day can be a major time commitment if the technique is to be done at its best.

ICSI is labour-intensive, and requires considerable training and experience. We find that embryologists may need many months before they get good results. It is very easy to damage the egg by inadvertent movement, and there is considerable skill in picking up the best sperm which are free from obvious defects. Clearly a very defective sperm will be incapable of fertilisation. A worry has always been that some sperm may be picked up which are in some way abnormal, but that the abnormality goes unnoticed. However, it seems that most sperm which are defective, even when the defect is not registerable under a microscope, are not capable of producing an embryo.

Once the eggs have been injected, they are returned to the culture oven. They are then inspected 20–24 hours later to see if fertilisation has occurred and to assess embryonic development. Embryos which show good cell development without too many fragments in them are suitable for uterine transfer. Those which are showing very good development – that is, with very few fragments (usually less than twenty per cent of the cells fragmented) can be frozen for later transfer if that is what the patient wants. Cryopreservation is not justified unless the embryo is showing good development with mostly normal cells.

Indications for ICSI:
- Men producing low sperm counts where less than 100,000 sperm may be capable of being retrieved for routine IVF.
- Men with very few sperm showing adequate movement. Men whose sperm show no movement at all may be unsuitable for ICSI, though certain genetic diseases causing immotile sperm (Kartagener's syndrome) may be suitable.
- Men with very abnormal sperm as seen under the microscope. When less than four per cent are normal, or where there are large sperm heads, ICSI may not be suitable.
- When high levels of sperm antibodies are present, and routine sperm-washing is ineffective.
- Repeated fertilisation failure during a previous IVF cycle.
- When there are limited numbers of sperm available – for example, in men who had sperm preserved in cold storage during cancer treatment and who are now sterile.

- Some men who cannot ejaculate normally – for example men with few sperm after retrograde ejaculation.
- Men who have damage to the tubing of the testicle (see page 75 on epididymal and testicular aspiration).
- Certain patients undergoing preimplantation for genetic defects (see page 83).

In addition to the indications above, ICSI may be considered in some couples where the infertility is unexplained and routine IVF has repeatedly failed. In these cases, there has usually been some indication of abnormal fertilisation, or lower than average fertilisation rates.

Results of ICSI (see also Chapter 7)

Probably the unit with the most experience in the world is that in Brussels, run by Professor André van Steirteghem and Professor Paul Devroey. They report that, in their hands in a very large study (using nearly 75,000 eggs) around nine per cent were damaged by the injection and could not be used. Approximately 72 per cent of ICSI injections resulted in successful fertilisation – a remarkable result considering that they were using abnormal semen, and that, in most IVF programmes using routine IVF only 50 to 55 per cent of eggs are fertilised naturally when the sperm are mostly entirely normal. Abnormalities of fertilisation occurred in about five per cent of injections. They were able to transfer at least one embryo in over 90 per cent of the cycles they treated, and about 22 to 29 per cent of transfers resulted in pregnancy depending on the indication for ICSI. Note that these figures are not live births per treatment cycle, but pregnancies per embryo transfer – nonetheless, they are stunning results.

It is clear that, in general, the results of the treatment of male infertility using ICSI outstrip the results from all other treatments by IVF. From being a condition with the worst prognosis, male sub-fertility has now become one of the most successful to treat. In Britain, in the most recent year of reporting 1996–7, 6,652 treatment cycles with ICSI were done and 21.6 per cent resulted in a live birth. In the same period, 26,868 cycles of conventional IVF were done and the live birth rate was 15.5 per cent. Of the 1674 pregnancies induced by ICSI in 1996–7, there were 229 miscarriages (about 13.6 per cent, which is roughly the normal miscarriage rate after IVF in most centres) and the number of stillbirths and neonatal deaths was just slightly lower than the average for IVF as a whole. These are immensely reassuring figures, because some people have irresponsibly suggested that the technology is being used at great risk to the children born.

The risks of an abnormal baby with ICSI

There are various theoretical risks associated with ICSI. They are:

1. Because the body's normal sperm screening process is bypassed, the operator may pick up a sperm which is genetically abnormal without recognising it.
2. The solutions to slow the movement of the sperm to allow the operator to pick them up in a pipette may in some way cause short- or long-term genetic damage to the injected sperm.
3. The act of injection may disrupt genetic material in the egg cell, causing chromosomal or other abnormality. It may also introduce extraneous material into the egg which would not normally be there.
4. Infertile men who need ICSI may have a genetic abnormality which they could pass on to their offspring.

If any of the above were true, one might expect to see a number of possible indications of increased risk. There might be reduced fertilisation rates, or reduced embryo formation. As we have seen from the Belgian figures, this is certainly not the case. Both fertilisation rates and embryo formation is improved by ICSI. There could well be a reduced pregnancy rate or possibly a higher miscarriage rate, both more likely when abnormal embryos are present. There is convincing evidence, both in Britain and elsewhere, that on the contrary, pregnancy rates are actually higher and that certainly the incidence of miscarriage is not increased.

A key observation would be the number of babies born with an abnormality. Again, the figures are greatly comforting. In Britain in 1998, 42 of the babies born after IVF had an abnormality of some kind (about 0.6 per cent of the total). Of these, six had an abnormality of a chromosome – mostly Down's syndrome – and the commonest abnormality overall, in twelve babies, was heart defect. This overall incidence is below the incidence of abnormality seen after normal conception in fertile couples. Thirteen babies with abnormalities were born after ICSI (0.9 per cent). This, again, is not higher than the national average after normal conception, spontaneous conception. The commonest abnormality after ICSI, in four babies, was a kidney defect.

The British figures are reassuring and fit in well with those across the world. Probably some 20,000 babies have been born after ICSI world-wide and the incidence of abnormality is certainly no higher than in the general population. It is true that a number of women have had pregnancy terminated after ICSI for major malformations seen at antenatal diagnosis. Once again, it is reassuring to observe that this major malformation rate is no higher than in the general fertile population. One can reasonably say that ICSI does not increase the risk of having a child with an obvious abnormality. However, there are some concerns about the possibility of infertile men passing on some long-term risk to their offspring.

The long-term risks of ICSI

So what about concern that children born as a result of ICSI may show abnormalities later in life? This slight concern is, as always, greatly fuelled by press speculation and by somewhat alarmist television reporting. It is necessary to examine the known facts. There is just one recent study of interest which was reported in *The Lancet* (May 1998). In Australia, Dr Jennifer Bowen and her colleagues examined children conceived after ICSI. They compared them with children born after natural conception or routine IVF. In all, 89 children conceived after ICSI were compared with 84 children born following routine IVF and 80 children conceived naturally. They took some care to ensure that the children studied were of similar birthweight and came from parents of similar age with a reasonably similar obstetric history. There were a similar number of twins in each group.

Children were followed up and assessed at one year old. Those born prematurely were assessed at a corrected age of one year. There was no difference in the health of each child, nor in the incidence of physical abnormality. The children, who were of course only one year old, were assessed for memory, their ability to solve simple problems, and their language skills. They were also assessed for motor skills.

Children born from ICSI showed no difference in general physical development or motor skills, but 15 per cent showed mild delay of mental skills. One or two children (the report is not very clear on this) showed rather more than mild developmental impairment. These findings are interesting but not, I think, alarming. The impairment was apparent in relatively few children and assessment has only been made at one year old. Most important to me was the fact that the authors of their paper record that significantly more parents of the group conceived by ICSI came from an unskilled occupation, and that one-third of the mothers and fathers of these children were born in a non-English speaking country. This was a statistically significantly greater number than the parents of the children from the other two groups studied.

Jennifer Bowen's data have not been confirmed by any other study. I have quoted it in detail so as to give the reader a proper background. The

Belgian team led by André van Steirteghem reported a study of twice the size (also in the same issue of *The Lancet*) – they examined 201 ICSI children and 131 IVF children at two years after birth, and compared them with children in the general population. They found absolutely no difference mentally or physically after ICSI or IVF. What I think is acutely interesting is that journalists reported Dr Bowen's findings in detail at the time of the reports in *The Lancet*, but most did not even mention that Professor van Steirteghem had conducted a larger study in older children. These are the very children who one might have expected to be more likely to show more pronounced retardation given that they were also one year older. This bias is, I am afraid, all too typical of many newspapers and television programmes reporting on the new reproductive technologies. There is no doubt that there is a large number of journalists out there just waiting to pounce. They claim to be offering responsible and important information, but they cause a great deal of unnecessary anxiety to many unfortunate infertile couples.

I am not saying that ICSI is free of all risk. The jury is out and it will be a very long time before we can be absolutely sure of its total safety. Nonetheless, the current evidence suggests no real risk at all, providing the infertile male is adequately screened before commencing ICSI treatment.

Screening the male partner before ICSI

Whilst in general the evidence is very much against ICSI predisposing towards damaged children, there is an important caveat. There are basically three categories of male infertility which may have some form of genetic basis. The sperm of these men may pass on some abnormality to a child born as a result of ICSI with one of their sperm:

1. Men with unexplained infertility are more likely to have a defect on the male (or Y) chromosome. It is known that the Y chromosome is abnormal in about thirteen per cent of men who are failing to produce any sperm at all, but who do not have any blockage of the tubes from the testis. Obviously men who are failing to produce any sperm will not be suitable for ICSI but a number of men who are producing very few sperm may have a similar defect on the Y chromosome. Such men are entirely healthy but presumably if their sperm are used for ICSI they are likely to pass on infertility to any sons.
2. Some infertile men – again those with apparently unexplained infertility – may have abnormalities of other chromosomes. They are particularly more likely to have a translocation which usually affects

two chromosomes. In one version of this condition, part of one chromosome is joined up with another. The female partner of men with translocations are more likely to have miscarrriages, but there may also be infertility. In some cases there may be a relatively normal sperm count, in others the count may be distinctly lower than normal. In addition to fathering a pregnancy which may miscarry, such men may also produce offspring that have abnormalities because of the chromosome defect. A particular problem is Down's syndrome, which is more likely with certain types of translocation.

3. Men with abnormalities of the epididymis, or of vas deferens, the main tube leading from the epididymis to the prostate gland, may carry the gene which causes cystic fibrosis. They are effectively carriers of this disease. This in itself does not matter, but if their partner also has the cystic fibrosis gene there is a one in four chance that any child may suffer from this disease. There may be other genetic diseases too, which are associated with similar abnormalities, but as they are bound to be very much less common than cystic fibrosis, the chance of the female partner having the same defect will be very much less. Consequently the chance of any child suffering some other rare genetic disorder inherited as a result of forcing fertilisation by ICSI is fairly remote.

With all the above inherited conditions, screening may be helpful. Any man considering undergoing ICSI, and having a low or abnormal count for reasons which are not clearly established, should have a blood sample examined. From this, his chromosomes can be cultured and a chromosome assessment or karyotype, can be made. In addition to looking carefully for any abnormalities of the paired chromosomes, an assessment of the Y chromosome can be made as well. Such a screen will not totally rule out the transmission of an abnormality which cannot be detected. It should, however, avoid any risk of Down's syndrome or other serious chromosomal defect in the offspring. Screening can also be done for cystic fibrosis. Given that this is a relatively simple test which can be done on cells taken from a mouthwash, such screening is to be recommended.

With these precautions, there should be no significantly increased risk of any child born as a result of ICSI having a serious inherited deformity. Obviously, some of the male children currently being born as a result of ICSI treatment may themselves have fertility problems when they grow to maturity. However, it seems to me that this is a bridge that can be crossed in twenty years' time – by when it is most likely that great advances will have been made in all these reproductive treatments.

Epididymal aspiration of sperm

A substantial number of men are producing some sperm in the testicle, but for various reasons few or none of them arrive in the ejaculate. Perhaps the commonest reason for this is surgical injury – usually men who have been sterilised by vasectomy and who may have had a surgical attempt at reversal of sterilisation which has not worked. It used to be thought that sperm from the epididymis would not be mature and therefore could not be used to fertilise eggs, but ICSI has changed that view. It is now possible to suck sperm from this very fine duct leading from the testis with quite a good chance of getting sperm which will be perfectly viable.

Epididymal aspiration of sperm may be indicated under the following circumstances:

- When there is congenital absence of the vas deferens, the main duct leading from the epididymis.
- In men who have had a failed reversal of sterilisation.
- In men who have had a failed operation to unblock the ducts of the epididymis, or men for whom it is thought that such an operation is not worthwhile. In most cases the primary cause of block is old, healed infection with scarring.
- Men who have no sperm in their ejaculate after repair of a hernia. It is presumed that in these men there has been some damage to the tubing leading out of the testicle.
- Men who have various conditions causing blockage of the epididymis where it joins the vas deferens.

The technique for epididymal aspiration of sperm is essentially the same as for ICSI. The woman's ovaries are stimulated to produce as many eggs as possible. Just before egg collection, the male partner is anaesthetised in an operating theatre and the scrotum incised. Some surgeons just expose the epididymis; others explore the whole testicle, temporarily removing it from the scrotum. The surgeon uses a microscope to identify the fine coiled tube of the epididymis. In most cases of obstruction the epididymis is dilated and therefore this is not a very difficult part of the procedure. A tiny incision is made in the tube as far from the testis as is possible. Although more sperm are likely to be found close to the testis, once the epididymis is cut it cannot be easily repaired; for this reason, the surgeon works back towards the testis in the hope of leaving some tubing for another attempt at a later date if required. A fine needle is then inserted into the cut epididymis and suction is applied with a syringe. Great care is taken to avoid getting blood into the sample because this can reduce the chance of fertilisation later.

Whilst the surgeon is doing this, an embryologist will have set up a microscope in the operating theatre, so the aspirated fluid can be examined for any sperm. If no sperm are seen, or if the motility of the sperm is very poor, the surgeon will make another exploration in the tubing, but a bit closer to the testis. If no sperm at all are found, the testis is replaced in its scrotal sac, and the surgeon may try to explore the opposite side.

Once sperm are obtained, the female partner is taken for egg collection. Eggs are collected by a needle inserted into the ovary through the vagina under ultrasound in the usual way, and then ICSI is done. Any spare sperm recovered may be stored in liquid nitrogen, where they will keep more or less indefinitely. However, frozen thawed epididymal sperm are never as fertile as are fresh sperm from the same source.

Recovery is usually fairly uneventful. The man will need to wear a tight bandage with a jock-strap for a week to ten days, but there usually is not much pain. The skin stitches that most surgeons put in are absorbable so that they do not need to be removed. Occasionally there can be some bleeding into the testicle after any surgical procedure of this kind. This can be very painful and unpleasant, but generally does not require any particular treatment beyond rest.

The results of epididymal aspiration are remarkably good. Most units report fertilisation rates close to those obtained with ICSI on ejaculated sperm. Usually the result is a bit less good, but pregnancy rates are very encouraging, and most IVF units achieve around a twenty per cent pregnancy rate after transfer of embryos in such cases.

Percutaneous epididymal sperm aspiration (PESA)

Some surgeons recommend percutaneous epididymal sperm aspiration (PESA). Rather then opening the scrotum and exploring the epididymis under the microscope, they prefer to use a needle which is stabbed directly through the skin, into the epididymis. Considerable claims are made for this technique, and there is no doubt that on occasions, with a certain amount of luck, it is possible to retrieve sperm after aspiration on a syringe. Sometimes this is done without a general anaesthetic with just some local anaesthetic in the skin.

The technique has the advantage of being simple and does not require a formal operation in the way that open surgery does. It has, however, a number of very severe disadvantages. It is, first of all, usually quite painful and the stab wound through the skin, though painless, in itself becomes very painful once the testicle is perforated. Many men who have experienced it are very reluctant to undergo it a second time. Secondly, it is not as reliable a method of collecting sperm. This is because the epididymis is a very small structure and unless it is considerable dilated it is very difficult to introduce a needle into it in this blind way. Thirdly, it is very common to get considerable bleeding where the needle enters the testicle and this can cause severe postoperative pain. Moreover, it can also cause scarring around the tubes and make any subsequent attempts at sperm aspiration very difficult, if not impossible. In our unit, therefore, we have abandoned PESA and prefer only to do open surgery for men with these problems. By doing an open procedure, one can explore the testicle and remove a small piece of testicular tissue for analysis. This is extremely useful because examination of the testicular tissue under the microscope can confirm that the testis is still capable of producing normal sperm. An examination of this kind (called histology) can also confirm that the testis is free of any serious disease which might be damaging to the man's health.

In practice, epididymal sperm aspiration can be repeated only a few times. After a while, the scarring prevents any further access to the epididymis and this is another reason why we do not favour the PESA procedure.

Testicular sperm aspiration

In a number of men, the epididymis is so badly scarred and the wall of this tube so thickened, that the only chance of retrieving any sperm is by collecting it directly from the actual tubules inside the testis itself. Testicular sperm aspiration is indicated in men with a very scarred epididymis and may also be used in some men who have a degree of testicular failure. Providing the testis is producing some sperm, however few, it may be possible to retrieve sufficient to allow an attempt at ICSI.

The procedure is similar to that of epididymal sperm aspiration. The man is taken to an operating theatre and, under a general anaesthetic, the testis is explored. A small piece of testicular tissue is removed from the testes and an embryologist examines this immediately under a microscope in the theatre. The tissue is carefully teased under a pool of culture fluid to release any sperm. This can take quite a long time. If no sperm are seen, another piece of testicular tissue can be taken and this procedure can be repeated a few times under one anaesthetic without any serious damage to the testes. Only small pieces of testicular tissue are needed, and, if necessary, both testes can be explored in this way. Pieces of testicular tissue can also be prepared for freezing. After washing in a suitable medium, they can be dropped into liquid nitrogen, in the hope that sperm may be retrieved later for a subsequent attempt at ICSI if the attempt with fresh tissue fails.

Remarkably, providing they are fairly mature, sperm taken from the testes have a very good chance of achieving fertilisation with ICSI. The results of fertilisation are not substantially different from those achieved with epididymal sperm. ICSI is not technically more difficult; indeed it may even be easier to pick up single sperm in a pipette because of their reduced motility. In our unit at The Hammersmith Hospital we have a pregnancy rate of around twenty per cent after this procedure.

Testicular sperm aspiration has the advantage that it can be repeated more than once in most men. It also has the advantage that a piece of testicular tissue can be looked at under a microscope after histological staining. This is important, because a number of men who have this kind of infertility may also have testicular cancer or testicular pre-cancer. There is an association between cancer of the testes and very poor sperm counts, and a testicular biopsy with proper exploration by the surgeon is a useful confirmation that there is nothing seriously wrong.

Findings indicating testicular aspiration may be futile

- When the blood level of FSH is raised. Testicular aspiration is rather less likely to be successful if the man has a very high level of FSH. This pituitary hormone is produced in increasing amounts when the testis is not responsive; this situation is exactly similar to that seen in ovarian failure. If this hormone is very high, it argues that the testes have stopped producing sperm and that there is more or less total testicular failure. However, in contrast to women, in whom a high FSH level is always very bad news indeed, some men are still manufacturing some sperm even when the FSH is raised. Consequently, there may still be some chance of finding sperm in the testes.
- When the testes are very small, soft and shrunken, as they are in many men with testicular failure, sperm manufacture may be faulty or totally stopped. Under these circumstances, testicular aspiration is much less likely to yield sperm. A testicular biopsy may be helpful to decide whether to proceed to ICSI based techniques.

- A negative testicular biopsy. If histology (microscopic examination of a small piece or biopsy of testicular tissue) of the testes clearly shows that no sperm are being produced and that there is total testicular failure, testicular aspiration is unlikely to be of benefit. This condition is frequently called arrest of spermatogenesis.

Spermatid injection

Some men may not be producing any mature sperm, but do continue to produce spermatids. Spermatids are immature sperm, the precursors of normal spermatozoa. There is a condition where the testes produce immature sperm but (possibly due to a genetic defect in many cases) the genes which control the final stages which mature the sperm properly are not being produced. In such men, in some units spermatids have been successfully injected into eggs, using the ICSI technique. Fertilisation has occurred and in some cases embryos have developed. In Britain, the regulatory authority (HFEA) has not as yet licensed the use of spermatid injections for human treatment. This is because it is thought that injecting a sperm which is so immature might risk the formation of an abnormal embryo which could lead to an abnormal child. Indeed, there are some recent reports which suggest that spermatid injection has given rise to the birth of several abnormal children.

Around the world, opinion varies as to the value of spermatid injection. Most serious workers feel that it is too experimental to be used and that in any case it will only give a very poor chance of pregnancy. For these men, therefore, donor insemination is probably a much simpler and wiser procedure if it is acceptable to them.

Alternative treatments not involving ICSI

There is no doubt that ICSI should not be used unless it is justifiably indicated. Even though it seems to be a completely safe technique it is foolish to use such a complicated treatment if there is a simpler solution. It is also relatively expensive. This is hardly surprising, given the cost of the equipment needed, the amount of space in a laboratory that is required, and the fact that considerable time needs to be devoted to it by a specially trained embryologist. There are a number of alternatives which patients may elect to use when undergoing IVF.

Mixing routine IVF with ICSI

In an attempt to avoid ICSI, some patients elect to have half the eggs that are collected treated by routine IVF. Quite reasonably, they feel that they want to try ICSI only as a last resort and they hope by these means to achieve natural fertilisation of sufficient eggs to create embryos for transfer. It is therefore quite a common request from some patients that their eggs are split into two lots and treated by two separate methods.

This is, I think, a satisfactory alternative. However, it does raise one curious problem which is still current at the time of writing. Rather ill-advisedly in my view, the HFEA have decided that patients should not have the transfer of a naturally fertilised egg at the same time as an ICSI fertilised egg. The reason for their insisting on this largely seems to be so that adequate data can be obtained on the fate of ICSI embryos. If a pregnancy occurs after a 'mixed transfer', they cannot clearly say whether the pregnancy has occurred as a result of natural fertilisation or as a result of ICSI – unless of course, the woman has twins; even then there would be no knowing which child was produced as a result of which technique.

Many people, like myself, feel that the HFEA view is far too heavy-handed over this issue. It seems to me that it limits the freedom of individual patients without any really good reason. We have been arguing the case with the HFEA for the last two years, and I think that eventually they may agree to change this ruling. At the present time, if a treatment does end up with one successful ICSI embryo and one successful naturally fertilised embryo, the patient has to have one of these two embryos frozen for later embryo transfer. As the freezing process itself will reduce the chance of a pregnancy one cannot but observe that this seems an entirely ridiculous, unsatisfactory state of affairs.

Percoll treatments

Some men with a rather reduced sperm count but with reasonably motile sperm can have the number of good sperm enriched. This is done by passing the sperm through a filtering medium. One filtering fluid which is widely used is percoll. It is a viscous solution which allows the best sperm to be concentrated for subsequent IVF. Once the sperm have been passed through the percoll, they can be collected and then placed in a tiny droplet of fluid medium. The egg can then be placed in this droplet and, because the sperm are concentrated around the egg, there may be a greater chance of fertilisation. A few units still use this technique because ICSI is not available to them, or simply because they or their patients want to avoid ICSI. However, the success rate with it is not nearly as good as that with ICSI. Percoll filtering is probably best used, therefore, merely as a diagnostic test to see if the sperm are capable of being satisfactorily concentrated.

Adjuvants to increase sperm vigour

There are a number of substances which have been used from time to time to make the sperm more active. These can be mixed with the sperm in the hope of making them more likely to fertilise the egg during IVF. The most commonly used drug is Pentoxifylline; another is caffeine. When mixed with sperm there is no doubt that these compounds can increase sperm motility. There is some limited evidence that they may also increase the fertilising capacity of sperm. However, various controlled trials have not clearly demonstrated the effectiveness of these drugs, and there is no evidence that there is a better pregnancy rate with their use. In consequence, very few laboratories now use these adjuvant substances.

Donor back-up

Because these complex and advanced techniques to enhance fertilisation may not work, it is worth considering having donor sperm ready as a back-up. In our unit we frequently arrange this if a couple wants it. If a donor is to be considered, it is most important that arrangements are made some weeks in advance of the IVF treatment. It really is most unsatisfactory to decide on a donor on the day of egg collection. Indeed, in some units, this may be refused because the appropriate advice and counselling has not been undertaken.

If donor insemination is being considered, it is wise for the man and his partner to get detailed counselling from a suitable expert who is familiar with the problems associated with donor sperm. It is essential to explore the family aspects of sperm donation and to review one's feelings about this very carefully. Once both partners are completely satisfied that they would be prepared to accept donor sperm if necessary, things can be taken to the next stage.

Once sperm donation as a back-up has been considered acceptable, a suitable donor should be found by appropriate matching between the donor and the infertile male. Appropriate donor sperm can then be held on reserve in the IVF laboratory depending on the outcome of sperm aspiration. It should be pointed out that once any sperm have been mixed with the eggs or once ICSI has been undertaken, it will then be too late to use donor sperm. One way around this problem is to separate some eggs for ICSI and to retain some eggs for exposure to donor sperm. A number of units do this but of course it does reduce the total number of eggs which are available for embryo transfer. Moreover, under the current rules of HFEA, embryos achieved by routine donor insemination cannot be mixed at transfer with those achieved by IVF and ICSI.

Emotional aspects of ICSI

One of the main problems with all these treatments for male infertility is that the brunt of the treatment falls largely on the female partner. The great majority of ICSI treatments are done with ejaculated sperm rather than sperm taken during an exploratory testicular operation. Even if the woman functions completely normally and the problem is entirely that of her partner, she has to undergo the extensive stimulation with drugs, the daily monitoring, the operation to collect the eggs, the embryo transfer and has the worry and the anxiety of waiting to see whether or not she is pregnant. She also takes all the risk involved with this complex therapy.

Remarkably, many women actually seem to prefer this. Others find it a very considerable strain. Some women feel that it gives them some kind of control over the whole process. I have frequently found that many women do everything to try and protect their male partner from the consequences of the infertility, and that this includes taking over all the burdens associated with treatment. Nonetheless, this can put considerable strain on a relationship, and a substantial number of men feel very guilty about the effort that their partner has made, or the risks which she is undergoing.

For all these reasons, I think that it is extremely important for these issues to be carefully thrashed out before an IVF treatment. We strongly recommend that all patients considering ICSI treatment, or indeed any complex treatment for male infertility, seek careful advice and consult an experienced infertility counsellor.

5
Preimplantation genetic diagnosis (PGD)

Introduction

A relatively recent advance in IVF has been the development of methods to screen human embryos for genetic defects. Preimplantation genetic diagnosis – that is genetic diagnosis in an embryo before implantation – is the first application of IVF for a condition other than infertility.

Most people born with a disease of purely genetic origin are likely to die as a result of it, and those gene defects which are not fatal usually cause severe disability. Genetic disease is extremely common. The list is both depressing and impressive. One in every 50 babies born will have a major birth defect, one in 200 will have a chromosomal defect. In Britain over 100,000 women are admitted to hospital with miscarriages each year, and the vast majority of this loss of life is caused by a genetic problem in the fetus. Most of these genetic problems are chromosomal. A quarter of children in hospital are suffering with genetically related illnesses. An eighth of adults in hospital have a genetic component to their disease. There is, for example, a genetic basis for much cancer, most heart disease, diabetes and some psychiatric disorders.

All single gene defects are caused by an abnormality in the DNA, i.e. the instructions held in the cell nucleus which determine the proteins made by our bodies, and hence most of our physical and mental characteristics. This DNA which is present in the nucleus of each cell in our body, can be regarded as a kind of code written in a language with just four letters. Each of these four letters represents one of the four chemical bases which are strung along the length of the DNA. The total length of the DNA in each cell is around 10,000,000,000 'letters' and the whole length of this DNA – the genome – can be thought of as a kind of encyclopaedia which gives the instructions to our cells. Each individual human has a slightly different encyclopaedia, which is why our inherited characteristics vary from person to person. The encyclopaedia – i.e. the genome – is broken up into 'volumes' – i.e. chromosomes. Humans have

46 chromosomes. Unlike the volumes of an encyclopaedia these chromosomes are arranged in pairs – 23 in total. One of each of these pairs is inherited from one or other parent. Twenty-two of the pairs are the same in males and females, but one pair – the sex chromosomes – is different. Females have two X chromosomes; males have one X and one Y. The Y chromosome, which determines maleness, is invariably inherited from the father.

The genes can be regarded as 'entries' in the volume of an encyclopaedia. Humans have roughly 100,000 genes. They give instructions for a particular body function. Some genes are 'read' every day – for example the genes which control the digestion of our food, or the way we move our muscles. Other genes may only be 'read' once in a lifetime – for example, the genes which control the implantation of an embryo in its mother's uterus – thereafter, those pages of the volume remain shut for life. Unlike a normal encyclopaedia, much of the lettering does not spell anything meaningful at all. The letters of this part of the DNA seem to be mere spacing for the genes which are in between.

Single defects result from a mutation – or misprint to continue the analogy – in the letters of the DNA somewhere along the length of an entry which spells out a gene. None of the genes are more than two to three million letters long; most are only a few thousand letters. However, a misprint of just one letter in a particular place can have a devastating effect. It can cause fatal disease from which there is no escape. Interestingly, a misprint in a place which does not spell out instructions for a protein will normally be totally harmless and unnoticed.

Defects in single genes fall into one of three groups:

1. The most common are recessive genetic defects. These will cause a genetic disease only when both parents carry a misprint in the same gene and pass that chromosome with that gene on to the child. Where both parents are carriers, the chance of any one child being affected is 25 per cent. There are about 4000 diseases caused by recessive gene defects. The most common in the UK is cystic fibrosis, which causes severe damage to the lungs and the digestive organs. Roughly speaking, about one in twenty of the population of this country carry the common recessive gene for this condition on one or other of chromosome number seven. The chance of a carrier meeting and marrying another carrier with the same gene misprinted is also one in twenty. Therefore, approximately one in 400 couples in the UK (20 x 20) are at risk of having a child with cystic fibrosis. On average one would

expect one in four of their children to inherit the chromosome with the defect from both parents. Thus the expected incidence of this disease in the population generally should be around one in 1600. This is confirmed by the actual, observed incidence in the British population.

Beta-thalassaemia is another recessive gene defect. It is a very serious blood disorder which causes severe and fatal anaemia. About 500,000 babies worldwide are born with this disorder. In countries like Cyprus or Thailand, the disease is so prevalent that it soaks up a huge proportion of the national health care budget. In Cyprus, as much as 60 per cent of all health care costs are related to patients with this terrible disease.

2. The second group of gene disorders are those caused by dominant genes. Any person inheriting one copy of such a gene from either parent will suffer from the disease. This is because a single copy on either of a pair of chromosomes is 'dominant' and will express the disease. It therefore follows that the parent carrying that gene will also have the disorder. For this reason, most dominant gene defects die out. This is because all gene defects tend to affect people from childhood onwards, and people with gene defects rarely live up to the time when they can reproduce and rear children themselves. Consequently, the dominant gene defects which are prevalent tend to be those which only start to show a disease process in older adults. A rare exception are those few dominant disorders which are relatively mild, allowing the affected person to have normal sexual relationships. The most important serious disorder of late onset is Huntingdon's chorea. It is a crippling neurological disorder which usually only starts to take real effect when a person is around forty. People with this disease start with quite mild symptoms of clumsiness, altered speech, forgetfulness or restlessness. By that time many may have had several children without knowing that they have inherited this defect. Once the disease takes hold, their bodies become rigid and bent, they have movements which they cannot control, and they start to become demented or psychologically abnormal in other ways. At the beginning of the disease they can often still work, but by the time the end comes, they require complete and total care in all aspects of their life. Death is frequently as a result of suffocation, but a number of individuals suffer so much beforehand that they commit suicide.

3. The third group of gene defects are those which are sex-linked. With very rare exceptions, they only affect boys. As described earlier, if the

baby's chromosomes are XX it will be female, if XY male. Some females carry a gene defect on one of their two X chromosomes but are normal in themselves because they have a 'back-up' X chromosome. But if a man inherits the defective X chromosome from his mother, the defective gene will be present and he will suffer from the disease carried on that solitary X chromosome. The chances of a man inheriting an X-linked disorder from his carrier mother are 50 per cent, an equal chance of inheriting one or other X chromosome.

There are about 300 known X-linked disorders. These include Duchenne muscular dystrophy, which causes the gradual onset of muscular paralysis in young boys. These boys get progressively weaker and are usually confined to a wheelchair by the age of nine or ten. They mostly die from suffocation in their teenage years, when they become too weak to breathe. Duchenne muscular dystrophy is common, affecting about one in 3000 boys in this country. Another sex-linked disorder is haemophilia. This is the bleeding disorder which affected the Russian Royal Family. It causes severe haemorrhage or bruising after very slight injury; the blood is simply unable to form a clot. These children get terrible joint disorders, because bleeding into joints is common. At the very least they require repeated blood transfusions and have to avoid many of the pleasures of life. In spite of great care, spontaneous unprovoked bleeding is common, and often one cause of death is sudden bleeding into the brain.

Requests for preimplantation genetic diagnosis (PGD)

Most families usually only find out that they carry a single gene defect when a close family member gives birth to a child with a specific gene disorder. Most of the couples we have treated at The Hammersmith Hospital have only discovered that they are at risk when one of their own children has already shown evidence of one of these disorders. Until recently, the only way carrier parents could prevent their having a second child with a similar disease was to undergo pregnancy screening by amniocentesis (removal of a sample of fluid surrounding the fetus) or chorionic villus sampling (removal of cells from the placenta for DNA analysis). They could then elect to have a termination of a relatively advanced pregnancy. In the case of many sex-linked disorders, the dilemma has been even worse. Because specific diagnosis of many sex-linked conditions is not always possible, parents can be faced with the decision to abort a male fetus without really knowing whether it is affected or not.

There is no question that termination of pregnancy is a very serious decision. Whilst many couples can cope with the loss of life that it implies, others find it quite devastating. But so often the only alternative has been to bring up a second child with a fatal defect. With a first child already terribly handicapped or dying, this is obviously a huge burden for very many couples in this situation. Termination of pregnancy leads many women, and some men, to feel permanent regret for the rest of their lives. There is a mixture of guilt and sadness which can pervade much of their lives inside and outside the home. Some women feel so badly about considering termination of pregnancy that they end their child-bearing potential by getting themselves sterilised. Quite frequently we find couples who live to regret that decision, as well.

Preimplantation genetic diagnosis (PGD) is one alternative for couples who cannot face a termination of pregnancy, or having once had the experience of termination are most reluctant to go through it again. PGD was developed in the late 1980s at The Hammersmith Hospital, and the first successful birth followed within a few years. Our initial attempts were really in the most desperate cases. It seemed that such couples had very little to lose by trying an alternative approach. One such woman was Julie. She carried the gene for Lesch-Nyhan syndrome, a disease which is sex-linked, affecting only boys. Julie had one child aged ten when I first met her. Her little boy, Peter, spent virtually all day strapped in a wheel-chair; he was incontinent and unable even to feed himself. He was strapped in the chair, because if his hands and arms were released his severe neurological condition led him to mutilate himself. I know of one such child who had bitten his tongue and most of his lips and finger tips away because of this compulsion; he eventually had his teeth extracted to try to prevent him injuring himself, but he still died of overwhelming infection caused by these injuries. These children have a severe metabolic disorder and develop painful kidney stones, and frequently die of renal failure.

Julie had had eight pregnancies; Peter was her only live child. All the others had either miscarried or been terminated because of the disorder. When I first met her she had decided that she would try anything rather than go through another termination. We elected to attempt PGD, by trying to select only embryos which were female for uterine transfer. Under these circumstances the worst she might expect would be a girl who might merely be a carrier of the disease. Julie's treatment was initially unsuccessful, although we were eventually able to treat her. Some three years after we first met, she had a healthy little girl. Just before this, we were quickly successful with two other very brave women who both carried different severe sex-linked disorders. They gave birth in 1990 after treatment – the first children born into the world after PGD.

Methods of preimplantation diagnosis

In families known to be at risk from inherited genetic disease, the woman is given ovulatory drugs to encourage the ovaries to produce a large number of eggs. These are collected through IVF and fertilised with the partner's sperm. In most units doing PGD, each embryo is cultured for two or three days until it contains about eight cells. One or two cells are removed from the embryo by microsurgery. Each of these cells is then broken up to liberate the DNA which can then be analysed. In the case of a recessive defect, the scientists can determine in a matter of hours how many copies of the defective gene the embryo has. If it has one it will be an unaffected carrier like its parents; if two, it will be affected by the disease; and if none it will be unaffected.

There are three basic ways in which an embryo can be screened for a genetic disorder before it implants in the uterus. The first two methods are now fairly commonly employed by nearly all units doing preimplantation genetic diagnosis. The third method is still experimental, but offers prospects for the future:

1. Analysis of the DNA from the nucleus of a cell removed from the embryo to identify specific single gene defects.
2. Evaluation of the chromosomes from cells removed from the embryo, using special staining techniques.
3. Examination of the proteins which are being produced by the embryo. A surplus or a deficiency may indicate a specific disorder.

Each of the above techniques requires the most exquisite laboratory control. In biological terms, it is still like an attempt at flying the space shuttle. Because the scientists are trying to detect DNA or chromosomes in single cells only, there is little room for mistake and the tests have to be extremely accurate.

Procedure

Initially, the couple are screened like any infertile couple undergoing IVF. Although few patients undertaking preimplantation genetic diagnosis are infertile, we have frequently found to our surprise that many couples who are requesting this technique have problems which might make IVF unsuccessful. It is surprising how often we find a problem with the sperm. Also, a number of women are found to have an abnormal uterus. Sometimes this is caused by a problem which occurred as a result of the previous pregnancy, for example infection or a curettage. In addition, older women requesting preimplantation genetic diagnosis may have hormonal problems which need careful evaluation.

Once the couple are scheduled for IVF, the woman's pituitary gland is suppressed in the usual way and drugs to stimulate ovulation are given. The aim is to try to collect a large number of eggs, without causing hyper-stimulation. As many eggs as possible are needed, because it is an advantage to have a really good number of embryos to study. Because some of the embryos are likely to have the genetic disorder in question, it is desirable to have plenty to choose from. There is then a greater likelihood of finding one that may be normal. Egg collection is done with ultrasound and then the eggs are taken in culture and prepared for ICSI. Single injection of sperm by ICSI is now done routinely in most cycles of preimplantation genetic diagnosis. This is because only by doing this can the team be absolutely certain that there is no contamination with more than one sperm. In the early days, when a cell was taken for DNA analysis, it was not uncommon for that cell to be surrounded by one or two extraneous sperm which had been left behind after attempts at fertilisation in the petri dish. The value of ICSI is that the team know for certain that only one sperm has been introduced into the culture and therefore there is not likely to be any contamination with DNA from stray sperm.

The embryos are now grown in culture. Early on the morning of the third day, the embryos are taken out of the culture oven and carefully inspected. Those which are dividing normally and which have regular cells in them are selected for preimplantation genetic diagnosis. At this stage of development, most embryos have around eight cells – ideal for PGD. Once the embryos have more than eight cells, the cells tend to stick together. This makes cell biopsy very difficult without risking damage to other cells. Removal of a cell from an embryo which has fewer than eight cells may result in too much of the embryo being removed, thereby destroying its viability.

The embryo is placed under a powerful microscope and is secured by a suction pipette held in a micromanipulator. This is very similar to the set up used for ICSI. A second micromanipulator is now used to introduce a fine pipette for drilling. In our laboratory, we fill the drilling pipette with a weak solution of acid and a tiny hole is drilled in the zona pellucida. This takes merely a few seconds to do, but requires considerable skill. Too much acid, and too much of the zona will be destroyed. Too little acid, and the whole procedure needs to be repeated. Once a hole has been made in the zona a wider bore pipette is introduced into the embryo itself and one, or usually two, cells are removed from the embryo. These are then immediately placed in special tubes which are closed very carefully to avoid the likelihood of stray DNA getting into the tube.

Each cell from the embryo is placed in a separate tube. The solution containing the embryonic cell is now alternately frozen and thawed, or treated in some other way to break up the cell. This fractures the nucleus of the cell which contains the DNA. Once the DNA has been released, it is then subjected to DNA amplification. The technique to achieve amplification is called the polymerase chain reaction (PCR). By using it, scientists are able to convert just one molecule of the DNA present in the nucleus of the cell, into several million molecules within the space of two to three hours. This is done by growing the DNA rapidly in the presence of enzymes, and by a process of careful alternate heating and cooling. PCR was first developed by Dr Kerry Mullis in California; he recently won the Nobel Prize for it. When he developed PCR, nobody (not even Dr Mullis) considered that eventually it would be possible to accurately analyse DNA released from a single cell. PCR, incidentally, has proved to be a most versatile technique. It can be used for a whole range of DNA analyses, particularly when DNA from a number of cells can be obtained. For example, it is used to diagnose viral diseases, for genetic finger printing in cases of disputed paternity, and the police may use it to analyse blood samples or semen stains in attempts to prove or disprove that a suspected person has indeed committed a criminal act. Readers may remember the case of O. J. Simpson in America, where the results obtained by PCR were used in evidence but the science-suspicious Jury didn't believe the evidence.

Once PCR has generated several million copies of the DNA, there will be enough for it to be analysed and stained so that individual genes, or parts of genes, can be identified. The particular defect in the gene, for example missing base pairs, can be compared with DNA from a person known to be normal. Thus diagnosis of a normal, affected or carrier embryo can be made.

Pains are taken to try to make the diagnosis on the same day as the embryo biopsy if at all possible. This then allows the doctors to return the embryos to the uterus on the third day after fertilisation. This is because, at the time of writing, embryos do not always survive particularly well outside the body for more than three, or at the most four days.

Once a diagnosis has been made, usually two healthy embryos are selected for transfer. It is our practice almost never to transfer more than two embryos. This is because in most families with affected children a triplet pregnancy would be a disaster. In general, it is difficult enough for them to cope with a twin pregnancy. Moreover, confirmation that the PGD has been done correctly and that the baby is normal is often requested. Antenatal amniocentesis or chorion villus sampling may be needed and it is easier to make accurate diagnosis in a twin or singleton pregnancy, rather than when there are triplets present.

The embryo transfer has to be done extremely delicately. This is because the hole in the zona pellucida makes the embryo more fragile, and there is always a risk of some of the cells escaping through the hole. This has happened several times in our experience, and it usually prevents the technique from working. Embryo transfer is normally done using an ultrasound machine to make certain that the catheter really is in the right place in the uterine cavity. Once the embryo transfer has been completed, the medical care is fairly routine. It is normal practice at around eight weeks to do careful scans, and an antenatal diagnosis is offered to couples after the eleventh week as a safety check.

The key issue immediately following DNA diagnosis is making the decision about which embryos to select. In a couple carrying a recessive disorder the overall mathematical probability is that one out of four embryos will be affected, one out of four embryos will be completely free of the defect, and two embryos out of four will be carriers. It is safest to put back only completely unaffected embryos. Of course, a carrier will be healthy and will not cause a problem in the child. However, there is a technical question about putting back embryos which are diagnosed as carriers. There is always the concern that a mistaken diagnosis may have been made. If a defect on one of two chromosomes has been missed the embryo may be thought to be a carrier, when it really is affected. If the embryo comes up with no affected DNA at all, at least there is an element of certainty that one chromosome is free of the genetic taint, and that, at worst, it is only a carrier.

At the time of writing, there are about eighteen or so different recessive genetic defects where PGD has been used in various countries. The commonest conditions are probably cystic fibrosis and beta-thalassaemia. Another disease for which PGD is being done is Tay-Sach's. This is common in Ashkenazi Jews and causes babies to die with severe neurological problems about the age of four years old. The diagnosis of sex for sex-linked disorders was also initially diagnosed using PCR. Now, with better developments in chromosome technology, identification of the X and Y chromosome are more usually undertaken (see below) because of the reliability of the chromosome staining procedure.

Chromosomal diagnosis

If a chromosomal diagnosis is contemplated, one or two cells are biopsied from the embryo and then the nucleus is carefully spread on a glass slide. This is a technically difficult procedure, requiring considerable expertise. As the nucleus is completely invisible to the naked eye it requires delicacy and precision not to lose the tissue. Once the nucleus has been obtained, it is treated by a method called fluorescent *in situ* hybridisation (FISH). With this technique, the DNA in particular chromosomes sticks to the DNA of a probe which has been labelled with a fluorescent dye. After incubation for several hours, the glass slide can be fluoresced using the beam of a laser under a special microscope. A bright coloration can be seen if a particular chromosome is present. At the time of writing, not all chromosomes can be examined simultaneously. So-called multi-coloured FISH can examine up to five, or at the most six chromosomes in one examination. This is sufficient for a surprising number of diagnoses. FISH is particularly useful for examining the sex of an embryo and it is very reliable. Stains are used which usually allow the X and Y chromosome to be very easily seen as brightly fluorescent dots. Normally, the Y chromosome is dyed pink and the X chromosome is blue. If there are two blue dots present, one knows that there is a female embryo; if there is a blue and a red dot, it is a male.

Just like DNA diagnosis by PCR, chromosomal evaluation is planned for completion on the same day as biopsy. In practice, the biopsy can usually be finished by early morning and the cells spread by mid-morning. It is therefore usually possible to get a chromosomal diagnosis between 5 o'clock to 7 o'clock in the evening and embryos can be immediately transferred.

More recently, FISH has been used to look for a variety of chromosomal defects. Gene defects are very serious, but chromosome defects are generally even worse. This is because a defective chromosome results in many genes being missing or abnormally active along its length. Most chromosome defects cause such severe abnormalities that the embryo is not viable. Others regularly cause miscarriage. A few are usually fatal to embryonic development, but some embryos with a defect survive. Chromosomal defects are most commonly of three types:

1. *Trisomies*. A trisomy is where, instead of there being a normal pair of chromosomes, there are three copies. It is thought that the three copies of a chromosome cause over-expression of gene products; possibly too much is as bad as too little. One notable example is Down's syndrome when the person has three separate chromosomes 21. This is occasionally compatible with life outside the womb. Only a fraction of embryos with trisomy 21 implant and survive to be born. When they do, they suffer from mental retardation, some have heart defects, and others problems with the bowel. Many of these children develop leukaemia.

   It is now just possible to screen cells from embryos for trisomy 21, and for several other trisomies as well. Some individuals are prone to have embryos with such defects. This is particularly true of older women, and some patients who have repeated miscarriages because of various ill-understood predisposing chromosomal problems. PGD is likely to be of value for them.

2. *Deletions*. Deletion of a chromosome, when one or both members of a pair are missing, is a very common problem. In most cases deletions are incompatible with life; an individual does need both copies of each pair of their chromosomes. An exception is Turner's syndrome, which is caused by deletion of one X chromosome in females. It is not invariably fatal, because there is a second copy of this chromosome present carrying the vital maternal genes. As it happens, over 90 per cent of embryos with Turner's do not survive and are lost by miscarriage or failure to implant. Those that are born are generally without proper ovaries, or have few or no eggs in their ovaries. They are therefore nearly always sterile, and generally menopausal. In addition, they often have some skeletal abnormalities and are frequently very short in stature.

   PGD can be used to see if both X chromosomes are present in certain women having repeated miscarriages, and those with unexplained embryo loss. This kind of screening may be helpful in future to try to understand why certain individuals are repeatedly failing to conceive after IVF and embryo transfer.

3. *Translocations*. Some people have part of one chromosome joined to another chromosome from a different pair. Providing there is no actual loss of genetic information, such translocations may be compatible with life. Indeed, many people with translocations are unaware that they carry them. They are otherwise completely normal, but may have more difficulty conceiving, or may have many pregnancies which

they miscarry. Translocations can affect men or women, and they may pass them on to their offspring, if they are fertile.

One common translocation which frequently causes repeated miscarriage is a mixture of one chromosome from pair 12 and 13. However, virtually any kind of translocation is possible, and they tend to be a unique configuration in each family affected. Tentative attempts are now being made to identify these defects in the embryos of some women who are repeatedly miscarrying. Much depends on where the 'break-point' is – that is the place where one chromosome breaks off and is joined to the other chromosome. To identify translocations, probes which identify DNA in the region of the break-point are generally needed. This requires a huge amount of work and is expensive to undertake. Nonetheless, it holds promise for the future.

Problems with preimplantation genetic diagnosis

Contamination

Contamination is probably the single biggest problem in DNA analysis. Because the scientist is dealing with one single copy of a gene (effectively a single molecule) it is all too easy to contaminate a sample. It is worth bearing in mind that a person coughing or clapping their hands ten metres away from the procedure will shed between thirty to one hundred cells into the atmosphere. One of these cells can easily enter the mix about to be analysed. It is also true that, even with meticulous cleaning, contamination is very difficult to avoid in glassware and pipettes. Although these are specially treated by acid solutions to avoid extraneous DNA, it is sometimes almost impossible to get rid of it. The handling of cells for diagnosis is done in a special hooded cabinet – this is first cleaned by destroying all stray DNA using fluorescent light. In spite of this, these hoods can become contaminated, and accurate diagnosis in single cells may then be impossible.

Failure of amplification

Sometimes the PCR technique simply does not work and insufficient DNA is amplified for analysis. There are various reasons for this. Sometimes there can be a technical failure of the PCR itself. Sometimes the cell or cells that have been removed at biopsy are abnormal, even though the scientist doing the procedure did not realise this at the time.

Moreover, some embryonic cells simply do not contain normal, representative DNA.

Biopsy of unrepresentative cells

Human embryos are frequently defective in all manner of ways. They may have abnormal cells, or they may have fragments of cells – oddly these abnormalities are sometimes eliminated by the embryo, which goes on to develop perfectly normally. Nevertheless these abnormalities almost certainly account for a proportion of those human embryos which often fail to implant. A single cell biopsy may inadvertently contain a cell or fragment that does not have a nucleus, or that has only an abnormal nucleus. Some embryos may be mosaic, with different pairs of chromosomes present in different cells. This can lead to wrong or confusing diagnosis. Alternatively, it is sometimes the case that the biopsied cells are undergoing cell death. All embryos may contain dying cells and these may also give a misleading diagnosis on analysis.

Damage caused by embryo biopsy

Before we started human embryo biopsy, large numbers of experiments were done with embryos from different species, including mouse, rabbit, pig, sheep and some monkeys. The findings were reassuring. Removal of one or two cells did not cause any fetal abnormalities and, in general, did not prevent further development. A considerable number of normal animals from different species were born safely after biopsy. Nonetheless, biopsy done inexpertly could cause damage to the embryo – the kind of damage that would be likely to be lethal to the embryo and prevent further development. Nonetheless, this is partly why the HFEA regulates this area of IVF very carefully indeed, and ensures the competence of those doing it.

Even when absolute care is taken by a fully trained individual, the embryo biopsy procedure itself can damage the embryo. Sometimes although the intention is only to remove one or two cells, other cells may slip through the hole produced by the zona drilling and the embryo disintegrates. Alternatively, the injury may simply cause the embryo to stop growing. This is not common. I find it remarkable that human embryos can be biopsied at all, apparently without any risk of harm on most occasions.

Considerations before PGD

Many couples are so desperate to avoid a termination of pregnancy that they are prepared to put themselves at ill-considered risk. It is most important that the following points are considered and talked through very carefully before going through preimplantation genetic diagnosis:

- *Failure.* Any attempt at preimplantation genetic diagnosis is much more likely to fail than to succeed. It will involve going through the whole panoply of IVF, with all the difficulty of stimulation with drugs and many hospital attendances. Even though people think they are more likely to succeed because they are normally fertile, we have not found this to be always true in practice. On average a single treatment by IVF has probably only about a one in four chance in establishing a pregnancy; PGD has slightly less chance because any affected embryos will need to be discarded. Therefore, anybody considering this technique must recognise that they will be doing something very demanding and that, in spite of all the commitment, it is still most likely to fail.

- *Miscarriage.* It seems there may be a slightly increased risk of miscarriage after preimplantation genetic diagnosis. Certainly, a number of the women we have treated have had an early pregnancy test which was positive but they did not go on to establish a proper clinical pregnancy. This, a so called 'chemical pregnancy', seems rather more likely after embryo biopsy than after routine IVF. At the time of writing we are uncertain whether or not miscarriage itself is also rather more likely. The usual miscarriage rate in naturally conceived pregnancies is about fifteen per cent. As around the world less than 200 PGD pregnancies have been successfully established, one would only expect to see 30 miscarriages if there was no extra risk. Two hundred pregnancies is too small a sample to say with any certainty whether or not miscarriage is likely to be more frequent. More experience is needed.

- *Twins.* Because we try to improve the chances of a woman getting pregnant, we normally put back two embryos. This, of course, carries a risk of twins; it is important for women undertaking PGD to recognise that their chance of having a multiple birth is increased. Triplets are avoided by limiting transfers to two embryos. But even a twin pregnancy can present special difficulties for many women in this situation. Couples can, if they wish, elect to have a single embryo transferred but this will reduce the chance of any pregnancy occurring.

- *Wrong diagnosis.* Because the methods of diagnosis are so difficult and because so many things can go wrong, it is not absolutely possible to guarantee that the diagnosis of freedom from the specific defect will be correct. It is inevitable that the analysis of single cells from embryos will be open to an element of doubt. Patients going through PGD should recognise that at best the technique only *reduces* their chance of having an affected child. We try to minimise this risk of a wrong diagnosis at The Hammersmith Hospital by doing various tests on embryonic and other cells beforehand. This is to ensure that our test procedures are as accurate as possible. We can normally refine the accuracy of diagnosis to around the 97 per cent level. This means that instead of having a four to one chance against having an affected child (as in the case with normal conception with a recessive gene carried by both partners) there will be a risk of about thirty to one against. Because there is still some small risk of having an affected baby, we generally recommend that patients consider either an amniocentesis at ten to twelve weeks after conception, or an amniocentesis at around fifteen weeks. They will then have a difficult decision as to what to do, but at least they are forewarned and can plan for the proper care of their baby after birth.

- *Inadvertent damage.* Extensive research has been done with animal and human embryos to try to ensure that removal of one or two cells does not cause harm. Of the 200 babies so far born, all are reported as being normal and free from abnormalities. There have been no reports suggesting that removal of a cell has caused defects in a developing fetus or in a baby after birth. However, in spite of all the positive evidence gained so far, prospective patients should recognise that the work is still experimental and that they are undertaking what is still an uncertain procedure. For that reason any child born after this work should be carefully examined and follow up should continue on a long-term basis to make certain that their development is normal.

- *Stress.* People undergoing preimplantation genetic diagnosis find that it can be emotionally demanding. All infertility treatment by IVF is, but there is something particularly poignant about trying to avoid a genetic defect in a baby. Many women who undergo this technique or who are considering it, have had a terrible experience previously. About half the women we have treated have already lost a child, the worst thing that can happen to any parent. They will have seen babies suffer, often greatly, from genetic disorders. Therefore they should be aware that IVF and PGD are really quite emotionally charged techniques. Remarkably, in spite of this, all but two of the women we have treated unsuccessfully have returned for a second or third treatment cycle.

One of the problems with PGD is the expense. At The Hammersmith Hospital we have tried very hard to keep costs as low as possible. Our view is that whilst this is a relatively experimental procedure it is not reasonable to expect patients to pay more than a minimal amount for it. In general, each treatment that we undertake costs us more than we feel that we can justifiably charge a patient. Most of the treatment we offer is free. At full prices, the procedures of embryo biopsy and genetic diagnosis on the biopsy itself probably add around £700–£1000 to the cost of each IVF attempt.

Future prospects

Plans are already well established to use PGD for those couples whose embryos are at risk of having disorders which cause disease in later life. Huntingdon's chorea (see page 85) is possibly the most important of these. Many people who will develop this condition do not know for certain that they carry this gene until they start to become poorly co-ordinated or lose mental capacity in early middle age. Another group of genes which cause disease of late onset are some of the familial cancer genes. They are generally uncommon but devastating. Typical is the familial breast cancer gene. Women with this gene are extremely prone to breast or ovarian cancer. Not only are they very likely to develop cancer in their thirties, many of these malignancies are hard to treat. They can grow unusually rapidly and may spread early to the other organs. Even if a women with this cancer is successfully treated by removal of one breast, it is not unlikely that another, similar cancer will develop in the other breast later. Some women, knowing they carry the gene even opt to have both breasts removed before any disease has manifested itself.

The gene for polyposis coli is a dominant gene and causes cancer of the large bowel. I know of some families where five or six members have all suffered this cancer by the age of forty-five. In one of these families, three people have died from it, one of them at the age of twenty-eight. Some forms of nerve cancer, such as retinoblastoma, are also inherited. A baby with of one of these genes is very likely to develop cancer of the eye by the age of two or three years. Even when one eye is removed because of cancer, often the other needs removal within a year or so. Even after this, these children are extremely susceptible to bone cancers, which are normally fatal.

One question that is sometimes asked is whether it is justifiable to offer genetic screening for embryos which if allowed to develop could live a perfectly healthy life. It seems to me that this is very much a matter for the families concerned. Providing their decisions do not greatly affect the society around them, their wishes and privacy should surely be respected.

Assessment of what the embryo produces

As outlined on page 88, PGD is done currently either by examining individual genes or by staining all or part of some of the chromosomes. The third option is as yet only experimental. Many of the genes which contribute to the function and health of an adult are already 'switched on' and active at the earliest stage of embryonic development. These genes are often producing proteins which may be detectable without even a biopsy of the embryo being necessary. It may be possible simply to test the culture media in which they are being grown, to see what chemicals they are producing.

One example of a typical chemical is the enzyme, Hypoxanthine Phosphoribosyl Transferase (HPRT). Absence of this vital chemical is caused by mutations in the gene responsible for its manufacture. Children who are born with a deficiency of the HPRT enzyme suffer from the disease Lesch-Nyhan syndrome, the disease which Julie (see page 87) carries and from which her son Peter suffered.

Attempts have already been made to detect the presence or absence of HPRT in embryo culture media. To do this, the embryo is grown in a minuscule microdroplet of medium – so tiny that if spilt, it does not cause a feeling of wetness on the fingers. After a number of hours of culture, the medium can be tested to see if HPRT is present; if not, it could be an indication that this embryo will suffer from Lesch-Nyhan disease. The great promise of this method is that it involves no surgery and no increased risk of damage to the embryo. With refinement, it should be possible in time to measure such chemicals as HPRT using automated machinery. This would eliminate much of the intensive work currently needed for both embryo biopsy and for chromosome detection. A major problem at present is that in the first few days after fertilisation, some of the HPRT present is from the mother. The cytoplasm of the egg – which is derived entirely from the mother – still contains some products from maternal genes, and this confuses these tests. At a later stage of development, all these maternal proteins will have disappeared. Therefore, one way around this difficult problem could be solved when embryologists are able to transfer more advanced embryos to the uterus – for example after five days when they have developed into blastocysts (see page 134).

Embryo flushing

Unsurprisingly, no woman relishes the thought of going through the whole panoply of IVF to obtain embryos to see if they are affected with genetic disorders. In several animal species it is possible to flush embryos out of the uterus at a very early stage and examine them. Might this be possible in humans too? This approach might just simplify the procedure of PGD. On the face of it, it would only require careful timing of ovulation and intercourse. Three or four days later, a tiny catheter could be placed in the uterus and the free-floating embryo might be retrieved for biopsy – or possibly placed in microdroplet culture overnight for chemical tests, before being returned to its mother's womb.

In practice, however, embryo flushing is likely to be much more difficult than it sounds. There is always the risk of dislodging an embryo and not recovering it. If the embryo was flushed into a fallopian tube by mistake, it could lead to ectopic pregnancy. The flushing procedure itself might be hazardous causing an increased risk of infection. And without superovulation – stimulation of the ovaries to produce many eggs – the examination of single embryos is going to be time-consuming and may need repetition over many cycles before a normal embryo could be identified. Many repeated cycles might be needed and for each attempt, a woman would require considerable day-to-day surveillance.

Polar body diagnosis

PGD can be done by examination of the polar body of the unfertilised egg. As discussed previously, all cells in the body have two sets of chromosomes which are paired. Egg and sperm cells each lose half their set of chromosomes before fertilisation. If this did not happen, the embryo would end up with too many chromosomes. Thus after fertilisation, the embryo starts life with its chromosome set re-paired, one half from the father and one from the mother. The polar body is a tiny piece of dead or dying tissue which contains one half-set of the chromosomes. It is extruded from the egg's substance just before the egg is matured for fertilisation. Once extruded, it has no further function and eventually disintegrates.

Using micromanipulation, the polar body can be removed from the surface of the egg. Polar body removal is no more difficult than embryo biopsy and has the advantage that, because it is done before fertilisation, it does not risk damage to an embryo. The polar body, once removed, can be stuck on a glass slide and its chromosomes stained using the FISH technique.

So, for example – if the polar body has no copy of chromosome 21, it is probable that both copies have been left behind in the egg. This process, called non-disjunction, is the usual cause of Down's syndrome. After a sperm fertilises such an egg there will be three copies of chromosome 21 – a trisomy. Thus screening of the polar body is theoretically helpful to avoid such a chromosome defect. If no copy of chromosome 21 was identified in the polar body, no attempt to fertilise the egg would be made – it would just be discarded. A certain amount of work has been done with polar body diagnosis, but my impression is that, at present, it is not very reliable. With more refinement it may be helpful, particularly in the screening of eggs from older women. They are more prone to non-disjunction and are therefore more likely to have failure of implantation, pregnancy loss or Down's syndrome.

6
The results of IVF

In vitro fertilisation is a much vaunted treatment, receiving huge attention both in the media and from patients. One could therefore be forgiven for supposing that it was incredibly successful. In fact, in the United Kingdom only a modest fifteen per cent of all treatment cycles end with a live birth. This success rate compares reasonably favourably with the success rates in other developed countries, in particular the United States, Israel, France and Australia which have some of the most sophisticated IVF programmes. So why the hype? On the face of it, a complex treatment which results in 85 per cent of patients failing does not seem so much cause for self-congratulation.

It is important to recognize, though, that one IVF treatment is only a single attempt to achieve a pregnancy in an isolated menstrual cycle. On this basis, it compares reasonably favourably with natural fertility in humans. The average couple under the age of around forty years old having reasonably regular intercourse will only have approximately an eighteen per cent chance of conception. Moreover, not all these conceptions will go to term, as some will miscarry. This chance of conception is improved somewhat by having very frequent intercourse in the same month. By comparison, IVF is not much worse than nature because it is only a single attempt at pregnancy.

The role of the Human Fertilisation and Embryology Authority (HFEA)

We are most fortunate in Britain in having a very efficient data collection system. In this respect, the Government's regulatory authority, the HFEA, is very much to be congratulated. It has devised a system of data collection which makes it very difficult for IVF units to report dishonest figures. No other country has a system which is as accurate. In this chapter, unless otherwise stated, I quote the official HFEA figures. Where the HFEA has not reported for a particular category of treatment, I quote the success from the computer records of The Hammersmith Hospital, usually over a period of four or five years. It must be remembered that the HFEA figures represent the national average – some units do better, others worse. The reasons for the wide variation in results are not so much due to the competence or skill of individual units. Rather, they very much depend on the kind of clientèle a particular unit is treating.

Results can be published in a great number of ways. The way they are reported has a considerable effect on how they are interpreted. The reported pregnancy rate is always higher than the live birth rate, not least because between seven to eighteen per cent of pregnancies will miscarry. Pregnancy rate per embryo transfer will invariably look more impressive than pregnancy rate per egg collection – not all eggs will fertilise, and not all fertilised eggs will become embryos. Pregnancy rate per egg collection will always look better than pregnancy rate per treatment cycle. So many patients start treatment but abandon it because they respond poorly, or because they produce too few follicles. It is actually possible for an IVF unit to publish its figures in such a way as to give the impression that it is twice as successful as a unit next door – even though the real success rate is the same in both units. The HFEA has insisted that all units publish their official data in a standardised manner, and they rightly require units to report the live birth rate per treatment cycle started. The treatment cycle is regarded as starting from the first dose of drugs.

UK success rates for IVF

Figure 6.1 shows British live birth rates for IVF, and multiple birth rates after IVF, over the last six years. The HFEA reports that there were just over 10,000 treatment cycles commenced in 1991. By 1996, the last year for which records have been published at the time of writing, there were

Figure 6.1 *British live birth rates for IVF and multiple birth rates after IVF over the last six years*

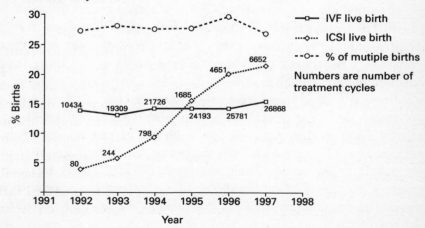

around three times as many treatments. IVF is becoming increasingly popular and acceptable. However, there are probably more than 600,000 couples in the UK suffering from infertility. A treatment which is only available to about five per cent of the affected population is one that is still inaccessible and highly exclusive – and this point, which is frequently missed is still the most important statistic to be derived from the HFEA's data. What will also be of considerable interest is that the live birth rate per treatment cycle has not improved very greatly in the last six years. Moreover, it is a worrying feature that the multiple birth rate has remained consistently at between 25–30 per cent. Multiple births remain a major concern because of the complications they cause. In Figure 6.1 the reader can also see the success rate for ICSI treatments. Unlike routine IVF, the success of ICSI has climbed sharply. In 1994 nine per cent of treatment cycles resulted in a live birth. The success rate is now 21.6 per cent and this success rate is such that it improves the overall figures for all IVF attempts.

Repeated attempts

The success rates for each successive treatment cycle attempted are recorded in Figure 6.2. Although this was once disputed, there is now no doubt that the best chance of having a successful pregnancy is during the first treatment cycle. The overall success rate is then 21 per cent, with a live birth rate of 17.4 per cent. One cause for optimism is that persistence is quite frequently rewarded. Remarkably, even when the eighth, ninth or tenth treatment cycle is undertaken, there is still a significant chance of a pregnancy. During the seventh cycle attempt the pregnancy rate is approximately 18.8 per cent. Thereafter it falls, and when a woman has had eleven or more treatment cycles the pregnancy rate per cycle is around eleven per cent with 8.6 per cent of cycles giving a live birth. At The Hammersmith Hospital, we have found that when women have persisted for five cycles or more, over 80 per cent achieve a successful pregnancy. But these figures do not tell the whole story. Clearly, most women do not go through ten treatment cycles. One prohibitive factor is the extreme cost of so many treatments. Another factor is the degree of involvement that such treatments require and the emotional demands that they make on the couple. But probably the biggest reason for discontinuation of treatment cycles is deliberate withdrawal due to poor prognosis. If the assessment during or immediately after an IVF treatment suggests a continued poor likelihood of success, it is responsible to dissuade patients from treatment. Consequently, the figures reported for

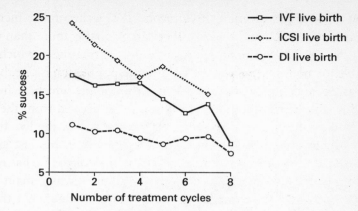

Figure 6.2 *Percentage success rates for successive treatment cycles*

repeated treatments may lead to over-optimism. Patients going through more than seven or eight treatments are generally those whose profile always suggested a good chance. They are self-selecting because of their youth, their ovaries respond well to the drugs, they produce a number of good eggs which fertilise and sometimes because they have already had one pregnancy – which makes another more likely.

Figure 6.2 also shows the success rates for ICSI for successive treatment cycles. In Britain, the overall success rate for the first treatment is a pregnancy rate of 27.6 per cent and this falls by the ninth treatment cycle to around 18 per cent. If one has the funds, and providing there are not too many adverse factors, it is worth persevering with treatment.

Results of insemination

One gratifying statistic has been the steady improvement in the success achieved with artificial insemination. Unfortunately, the results of intra-uterine insemination using the male partner's semen are not recorded and reported. But we do have the results for donor insemination cycles and they are likely to be somewhat similar. Because non-donor cycles do not use frozen, stored sperm, the results for them are actually likely to be better.

According to the HFEA records, about 5419 patients received donor insemination in 1996–7. The records, as reported, make it unclear as to the precise number. We do know that there was a total of 14,333 cycles, however – a few were done using GIFT. A slight deficiency in the HFEA report is that it does not state exactly how many GIFT cycles with donor sperm were done, but it is likely to be very few – probably around 50. The total number of DI cycles resulted in 1661 clinical pregnancies, and

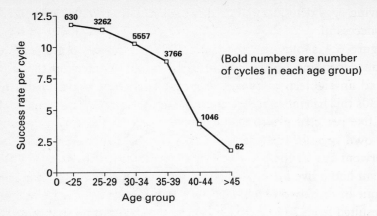

Figure 6.3 *The results of DI by age group*

203 miscarried (about twelve per cent). Another thirteen were ectopic pregnancies (about 0.8 per cent) – probably equivalent, incidentally, to the general incidence in the average population. Some 1373 live births resulted which is an overall success rate per cycle of 9.5 per cent. The success rate was almost one per cent better if the cycles were stimulated with drugs. These excellent figures show that DI has consistently improved since 1991, when the live birth rate was five per cent. In the last four years the number of donor cycles carried out in the UK has dropped by around 70 per cent – this is almost certainly due to the introduction of ICSI. Figure 6.3 shows the results of DI by the woman's age. It is not entirely safe to assume that the results of IUI using a partner's sperm would be similar. This is because there may additional infertility factors (particularly in older women undergoing IUI with a partner's semen) which reduce the chance of pregnancy.

Factors which may influence success

Age

The biggest single factor affecting IVF outcome is the age of the female patient. Women are born with all their eggs in the ovary, around 2,000,000 eggs at the time of birth. By the time a girl reaches puberty she has perhaps only 300,000 eggs left in her ovaries. Thereafter, although she is only ovulating one egg each month (approximately 400 eggs ovulate during an average reproductive lifetime), by the time she reaches her menopause she has very few eggs left at all. The number of eggs in the ovary is rapidly diminishing because they die off. It is also thought that surviving eggs deteriorate. For this reason, IVF in older women is much less successful.

Figure 6.4 shows the results for 1996–7 for all IVF treatments in Britain depending on the age of the woman. Women up to the age of 32 had an eighteen to twenty per cent chance of a live birth. By their mid-30s this has fallen to below fourteen per cent. After the age of 40 less than five per cent of women achieve a successful live birth when using their own eggs. In the last year when reports are available, 202 women underwent IVF at the age of 45 or over using their own eggs. Only two of them had a live birth. In the same period of time 32 women had ICSI and one of those women had a live birth. A total of only three babies, in all, resulted from 234 treatment cycles. It is also certain that these women had more costly treatment, because women over 40 often require four or five times the amount of FSH compared to women in their early 30s. The extra cost can be as much as £1500 in drugs alone.

There can be little doubt that this reduced fertility is mostly due to poor ovarian performance, and to poor egg quality. Although the uterus may be a bit less receptive in older women, the results of egg donation confirm that egg quality is the biggest factor. When an older woman receives an egg taken from a woman under the age of 35, the pregnancy rate is consistently high. The high miscarriage rate in older women also implies a problem with egg, and therefore embryo, quality. Women over 44 have almost a 50 per cent chance of miscarriage when they conceive with their own eggs. When they are recipients of donor eggs, their chance of miscarriage is only slightly above average.

Figure 6.4 *The results for 1996–7 for all IVF treatments in Britain*

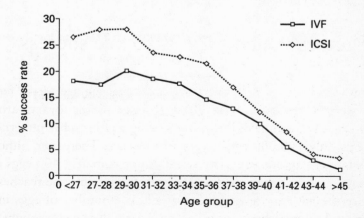

Number of embryos transferred

A second factor which influences the chance of success is the number of embryos which are transferred. Interestingly, women who produce large numbers of embryos during a single treatment, whether they have them transferred or not, also have a better chance of a successful outcome. Perhaps the number of embryos produced is related to ovarian responsiveness, and thus to embryo quality.

Figure 6.5 shows the UK success rates for women having two or three embryos transferred. The pregnancy rate per treatment cycle increases with the number of embryos transferred but the overall live birth rate is not greatly altered. Note that the multiple birth rate is significantly higher when three embryos are transferred and over one-third of patients have a twin pregnancy. In young, comparatively fertile women the multiple pregnancy rate is over 40 per cent. In my view this is completely unacceptable. In Britain last year no fewer than 222 patients had a triplet or quadruplet pregnancy. This is a desperately serious, unhappy situation. Many of these babies do not survive and the ones that do require intensive care with a long time in an incubator. It has been calculated that it may cost between £30,000–£45,000 to keep one baby from a triplet conception in an incubator. This implies a horrendous cost to the health service. Moreover, not all these babies survive completely intact. Approximately ten per cent of them may show some form of brain damage, and many others will have some other form of handicap. There is little doubt therefore that ideally the number of embryos transferred to the uterus should be limited.

Figure 6.5 *UK success rates for women having two or three embryos transferred*

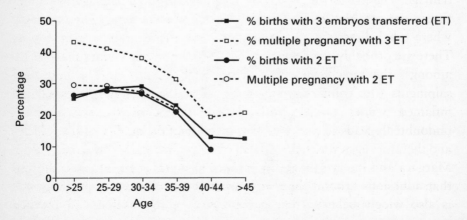

Cause of infertility

Until recently, the HFEA refused to accept what large clinics like our own were telling them – namely, that the cause of the infertility had a powerful affect on success rates. The latest figures published by the HFEA itself now leave no room for doubt. Indeed, the real differences between success rates for different causes of infertility are even greater than reported. This is because many units have a poor record of investigation. They frequently have not clearly established the cause of infertility. Moreover, the IVF data collected by the HFEA do not take account of all the important causes, for example infertility caused by uterine disease, failure of ovarian responsiveness, or infertility caused by two or more factors working together.

Now that ICSI has become firmly established, there is no doubt that IVF for male infertility is by far the most successful treatment. Between 20–25 per cent of patients across the country achieved a live birth in 1996-7. In females, treatment of mild endometriosis gives the best chances of success. Unfortunately, the HFEA figures do not distinguish between mild, moderate and severe endometriosis. There is a huge difference in results; at The Hammersmith Hospital, patients with severe endometriosis have a relatively low success rate; less than 50 per cent of that achieved by patients with superficial endometriosis.

Women with ovulatory infertility do well, but the prognosis depends on the cause of failure to ovulate. Polycystic ovarian disease is generally associated with a better outcome providing the patient is not overweight. Patients who ovulate only poorly with stimulatory drugs fare much less well.

The worst common category of infertility is undoubtedly tubal damage. The live birth rate for the treatment of tubal damage was under fifteen per cent nationally during 1996–7. In some units, like our own, where tubal disease is particularly bad, the success rate is even poorer. There are probably several factors which make patients with tubal disease amongst the most difficult to treat. Firstly, patients who have had salpingitis (the commonest cause of tubal damage) mostly have had inflamed ovaries as well. Inflammation of the ovary, or oophoritis, undoubtedly leads to scarring. This may affect the quality of the follicles and therefore eggs which are produced. Experimental work done by Raul Margara and me at The Hammersmith Hospital years ago also showed that adhesions around the ovary decrease the chances of pregnancy. It is also widely believed that patients with a hydrosalpinx (a blocked fallopian tube full of fluid) are rather less likely to conceive. Possibly the fluid in the tube may, in some way, impair the implantation process. A further factor is that many women who have had tubal inflammation have some damage in the uterus as well.

Uterine causes of infertility are not even recorded by the HFEA. This is because far too few units really assess the uterus properly. Uterine investigation is poorly done and poorly understood even though this is where the baby, if successfully implanted, will grow. Uterine damage is likely to affect the chance of implantation, and may also increase the risk of miscarrying. Following tubal inflammation, adhesions in the uterus are more common and changes in the muscle wall of the uterus are more frequent. Women with multiple fibroids, or a single fibroid indenting the uterine cavity, undoubtedly have a reduced chance of success after embryo transfer. Indeed a fibroid inside the cavity of the uterus may act rather like a contraceptive coil, preventing implantation. Another uterine defect which certainly decreases the chance of implantation is congenital deformity. Patients who have a uterus wholly or partly split into halves as a result of a birth defect are much more likely to have difficulty with conception. The good news is that both fibroids and these congenital defects can be easily treated before IVF. The treatment of intrauterine adhesions is also important (see Chapter 2). Most uterine adhesions follow inflammation after pregnancy or after a termination of pregnancy. Many of these patients can be simply treated and the uterine cavity cured of the major defect. In my view, to transfer embryos into a cavity which is badly damaged without knowing it, is close to being negligent.

There are a number of other categories which will make the chance of success less good. Women with severe ovarian disease are rather less likely to produce eggs. This includes women who have persistent cysts or those women who have had regular operations to remove multiple cysts from the ovary. Such cysts on the ovary should not be confused with polycystic ovarian syndrome which has a good prognosis. It is patients with pathological cysts which damage the substance of the ovary who are less likely to conceive. The same is also true for those women who have endometriotic cysts on the ovary with extensive fibrosis and scarring. Sadly, extensive endometriosis tends to reduce the total substance of the ovary and it frequently results in rather poor response to ovulation. In addition, women with extensive ovarian disease sometimes experience a slightly earlier menopause than average, because so much ovarian tissue has been destroyed.

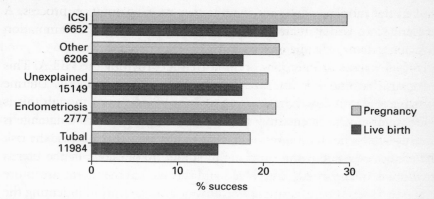

Figure 6.6 *Percentage of women with pregnancy and live births*
Taken from HFEA data for 1996–7. Note that numbers of cycles (under cause) does not add up to 33520 (the total number of cycles done in that period) because some patients had more than one cause reported

What to my mind is most interesting about Figure 6.6 is that it shows that much IVF is being done almost without any real idea of the diagnosis. 33,520 cycles were done but 42,768 causes are listed, some patients (28 per cent) having more than one cause for their infertility. This, in practice, is far too low a figure – in an average IVF clinic, one would expect 35 to 40 per cent of women to have a dual cause for their problem. Also, infertility caused by polycystic ovaries or failure to ovulate is not listed at all – presumably they come under the category 'other'. But even if the maximum of 6206 patients had anovulatory infertility, this would only be around fourteen per cent, which seems a low incidence. Over one-third of patients were in the 'unexplained' category; this again suggests inadequate attempts to arrive at a diagnosis.

Adenomyosis

I have separated adenomyosis from other uterine disease because of its special nature. Adenomyosis is a disease where the lining of the uterus grows into its wall and causes scarring. It is more common in older women and more common in women who have a history of endometriosis. Many women with adenomyosis have painful periods, and the pain characteristically usually starts before the onset of menstruation. They may also have rather irregular bleeding and sometimes there is prolonged spotting immediately before or immediately after a period.

Scarring like this in the uterus undoubtedly decreases the chance of an embryo transfer being successful. The precise mechanism by which adenomyosis interferes with infertility is not clear, but research by Dr Jan

Brosens at The Hammersmith Hospital suggests that it may interfere with the natural motility of the uterine muscle and may result in difficulty in implantation. Unfortunately, adenomyosis can be diagnosed but is very difficult to treat. The diagnosis can be characteristically made on a good quality hysterosalpingogram, or occasionally by magnetic resonance imaging. Treatment is less satisfactory and, although it is sometimes possible to damp down the scarring process by administering hormones, there is not much evidence that this will improve the chance of an embryo transfer working. Our impression is that significant adenomyosis decreases the chance of a successful outcome by about 50 per cent, depending on how much of the uterus is involved and the age of the patient.

Poor ovarian response

One of the biggest problems in IVF is poor ovarian response. A number of women simply do not respond to the stimulatory drugs. They produce fewer follicles than average and the follicles tend not to contain a properly mature egg. Sometimes the eggs show various cellular abnormalities when they are collected and often they have a lower than average fertilisation rate. When an embryo is produced, such women tend to have a reduced chance of it implanting successfully. The cause of poor ovarian response is not understood. Undoubtedly, in many women it is due to an earlier than average aging process. Poor ovarian response is much more common in women in their late 30s and very early 40s, than it is in young women. However, it is not uncommon to see the same phenomenon in a woman around or after the age of 30. Such patients have a poor chance of success at IVF, and need to be warned of this in advance before going through repeated treatment cycles. Unfortunately, although a number of tests of ovarian response have been devised, none is a particularly accurate predictor of the likelihood of a poor response. Various tests have been tried, including giving a woman a weak dose of FSH, or a small dose of clomiphene. Other women are given a single shot of Buserelin and the body's response measured on ultrasound and the level of oestrogen in the blood is also measured.

Previous pregnancy

Results at The Hammersmith Hospital clearly show that those women who have had a pregnancy in the past are more likely to be successful at IVF. What is of interest is that the history of a previous pregnancy is more important than the nature of the pregnancy – whether it failed or succeeded. Our figures suggest an extra chance of almost 30 per cent in women who had been previously pregnant. Patients who had a live birth or a miscarriage were almost as equally likely to be more successful after IVF. Patients who had previously had an ectopic pregnancy were only slightly less well-off. Even patients who have had a totally failed, very early pregnancy were statistically more likely to have a successful outcome if they underwent a further treatment cycle. Such so-called biochemical pregnancies, when the level of HCG – or pregnancy hormone – rises to perhaps no more than ten or twenty units in the blood stream are common after IVF. They can be devastating because women initially feel they have succeeded. But at least there is the knowledge that even a weakly positive biochemical pregnancy indicates it may be worth trying another treatment cycle.

Duration of infertility

Women who have been infertile for a long period of time are less likely to conceive after IVF. In our unit, patients who have been infertile for more than seven years have about half the chance of successful conception after IVF. This effect is not due to age as even younger women (under 35) showed a significant worsening in success the longer they have been trying. This is a distressing statistic but it should not, in itself, prevent a person trying IVF treatment. The statistic probably has more implications for IVF units than it does for patients. In units like ours, which treat the hardest cases, attempting to help women who have been infertile for very long periods is bound to depress the clinic's success rate.

Difficult embryo transfer

It is not uncommon to have considerable difficulty in transferring the embryos to the uterus. Sometimes the cervical canal is distorted or very curved, and it is a real problem for the doctor to get the catheter round the bend and into the uterine cavity. Sometimes repeated attempts at embryo transfer have to be made and it is not unusual for such transfers to be extremely uncomfortable. On occasion, the transfer can draw blood from the cervix and on rare occasions from the inside of the uterine cavity. At The Hammersmith Hospital, to give ourselves confidence that we are transferring the embryos correctly, we use the ultrasound machine. The catheter loaded with the embryos is placed through the cervical canal, and simultaneously another doctor places the ultrasound probe over the bladder of the patient, on the abdominal skin. It is thus possible to see the outline of the uterine cavity and the tip of the catheter. Immediately the fluid containing the embryos is released into the cavity, a bright glow can be seen on the ultrasound screen. This is evidence that the embryos are almost certainly in the right place.

A number of studies have been done to assess whether the quality of the embryo transfer clearly alters outcome of treatment. Results are disputed, but most research studies do not confirm that a difficult transfer or an easy transfer makes much difference. Clearly it is important that the embryos are in the right place, but the length of time that the transfer has taken, the amount of discomfort that the embryo transfer has caused, and the number of times that the catheter has to be changed before transfer does not seem to change the prognosis. Bleeding from the cervix does not effect the outcome. However, two trials (including one from The Hammersmith Hospital) do suggest that if there is uterine bleeding from the cavity itself, the chances of a pregnancy may be reduced.

For this reason, we have long advocated that all women undergoing IVF have a dummy embryo transfer about one month before the actual treatment. At The Hammersmith Hospital, at an initial coordinating clinic, a fine catheter is placed through the cervix in a mock attempt at embryo transfer. If there is any significant difficulty, the patient is then reassessed. If there is further difficulty, then during the month of treatment or just before it, a quick anaesthetic is given and the cervix is dilated with metal probes. This makes it easier to perform an embryo transfer on the actual day, when it is vital to get the embryos in the right place. On occasions, when the cervix is extremely distorted or abnormal, it may be justified to do the embryo transfer under a general anaesthetic. Patients sometimes worry that general anaesthesia may adversely influence an early pregnancy, or may reduce chances of implantation. There is no evidence for this.

Frozen embryos

The results of frozen embryo transfer are considerably less successful than those achieved in fresh cycles. Embryo freezing certainly destroys some embryos; others do not survive the thawing process. When, after this process of attrition, remaining embryos are transferred, only about 11.6 per cent result in a live birth, or approximately half that achieved with fresh embryo transfer.

Ovarian stimulation

IVF done without stimulation is less successful. One or two British centres have been conducting IVF using natural cycles. The ovaries are not stimulated with superovulatory drugs at all, or only just with a tiny dose of clomiphene. Sometimes a dose of HCG is given to trigger ovulation. But the inconvenience to patients is not negligible. Cycles have to be tracked to time egg collection, and regular ultrasound and blood sampling is needed. Once ovulation is imminent, a single egg (usually) is collected by needle puncture.

In total, during 1996–7, 144 women underwent 151 treatments without stimulation. On 49 occasions it was possible to achieve an embryo transfer; four women had a live birth afterwards. Two of these women had a set of twins. The overall success rate was 2.6 per cent – only one tenth of what can be achieved when the ovaries are stimulated. Therefore, probably the only indication for unstimulated IVF cycles is when a donor egg or embryo is used, or possibly if there are religious objections to collecting several eggs simultaneously.

In the same year, 764 patients had a total of 817 cycles using a donated egg or donated embryo without stimulation. Of these treatments 22.2 per cent resulted in a live birth and a total of 249 babies were born in all – a number of them having twins.

Stress

Many women believe that the stress they experience during each IVF attempt causes them to fail to become pregnant. This concern is hardly surprising. It is well known that stressed animals frequently have reproductive problems. Cattle or horses who are badly stressed have a lower than average pregnancy rate; cows who are undergoing stress have diminished milk yields. For many years, I kept rabbits for various breeding experiments. These lovely animals always looked happy and contented, but when on occasion there was noise where they were housed they looked stressed. When the rabbits were unhappy there was no question that the ovulation rate was poorer, and the number of baby rabbits that they produced was lower.

The mechanism in humans, however, is a good deal more complicated. In many extremely stressful situations women still retain fertility. At The Hammersmith Hospital, an extremely careful study of stress and infertility was made a few years ago by my colleague Dr Enda McVeigh. He, together with Professor Susan Golombok of City University, designed a detailed and statistically valid questionnaire which IVF patients were requested to complete before, during and after IVF treatment. This scored their stress levels extremely carefully, using well-accepted psychological parameters. Dr McVeigh also took numerous blood samples from these patients to measure various hormones associated with stress. This part of the study was done in collaboration with Dr Vivette Glover. The measurements included the levels of hormones coming from the adrenal gland (the so called fight and flight hormones) and various brain hormones, including endorphin levels which are altered during stress. After detailed analysis, we could find no evidence of any difference between those women who had a successful outcome and those who did not. Moreover, women with a known cause for their infertility were not substantially different from those with unexplained infertility. Our conclusion was therefore that stress does not cause unexplained infertility nor does stress clearly adversely effect the outcome of IVF. However, it was clear that unexplained infertility did cause stress and that undergoing IVF, not surprisingly, also caused considerable stress.

Rest after embryo transfer

Not surprisingly, women who have had an embryo transfer feel fragile and very worried about exertion. They feel that the slightest knock, or fall, may in some way dislodge the embryo developing in their uterus. Other women are very worried about moving from the couch after the embryo transfer has taken place. They are very concerned to lie still for as long as possible.

Several studies have been conducted, and the general results suggest that it makes no difference what you do after an embryo transfer. It is almost certain that there is no way a normal embryo or a normal pregnancy can be dislodged by jumping around, by a fall or by physical work. Rest immediately after embryo transfer does not appear to make any significant difference either. One recent study compared women who were lying on a couch for 30 to 60 minutes after transfer with those who were asked to move within fifteen minutes. The pregnancy rate was the same in all groups. Nevertheless, for purely psychological reasons it may be unwise for clinics to move their patients too soon after embryo transfer. For this reason we encourage women to lie reasonably still after it for 30 minutes or so.

Obesity

Patients who are very overweight have a significantly reduced chance of pregnancy. This depressed chance affects virtually all forms of infertility treatment. It is particularly true for IVF. Patients who are very overweight almost halve their chance of success. What is not clear is whether or not patients are less likely to become pregnant whilst they are attempting to reduce weight, and therefore on a reduced diet. The evidence is rather equivocal. We try to persuade obese patients to try to lose as much weight as possible before entering the IVF programme. On the whole it is probably better to start treatment once dieting has been completed and the weight becomes stable.

Smoking, coffee drinking and other sins

There has been a great deal of rather anecdotal evidence which suggests that smoking is harmful to the outcome of IVF. A number of papers published in scientific journals have suggested that smokers produce fewer eggs and embryos. However, the evidence that they have a reduced pregnancy rate is not as good. It is true that women who smoke heavily are more likely to have an earlier menopause, and therefore may produce fewer eggs later on in reproductive life. Some years ago, Dr Liz Sheriff did a study in our unit and compared smokers with non-smokers. She could find no evidence that smoking made a substantial difference to the successful outcome of IVF. It was true, however, that women who were giving up smoking at the time of IVF did significantly less well when they went through a treatment simultaneously.

It would seem that Dr Sheriff's study should be repeated. Other workers in my unit are currently measuring the levels of nicotine metabolites in the ovarian follicles, found at the time of egg collection. Smokers certainly show marked increases in these chemicals. Our impression is that they may adversely affect the egg. It would be interesting to see whether they also adversely affect the chance of pregnancy.

It is known, however, that smoking definitely affects male fertility. Men who have rather poor sperm function or decreased sperm production undoubtedly do far less well if they are still smoking heavily. They should be encouraged strongly to stop smoking if they are contemplating any form of reproductive treatment. It seems stupid to put their wives through the stress of IVF and possibly ICSI, if they are undermining the chance of treatment working optimally.

Coffee and tea drinking have been blamed for the failure of IVF. I know of no good studies which show convincing evidence. It has also been suggested that alcohol may reduce the chances of IVF working. I feel that this is almost certainly not the case. Some years ago, Stephen Hillier (now Professor at Edinburgh University) and I conducted a study giving women a glass of wine at the time of embryo transfer. This was done mostly to calm them down and to help relax the uterus. It was also true that at that time we did our transfers at the end of the day, and we were more than happy to relax with our patients. We found that rather than reduce the chance of a pregnancy, a glass of wine seemed to actually improve the chances of our patients becoming pregnant. It was our impression that a glass of good red wine was slightly more effective in this respect than a glass of white. There was no difference in wine produced in France from wines from Germany, or even Chile.

7
Adjuncts and improvements to IVF

Better drugs to stimulate ovulation

As we have seen, follicle stimulating hormone (FSH) and luteinising hormone (LH), the hormones used to stimulate the ovaries to mature and then release eggs, are normally produced by the pituitary gland. Until recently these hormones were extracted from the urine of menopausal women. One disadvantage of using such biologically derived drugs is that the body treats them as a foreign intrusion and when they are given to another woman, antibodies can be formed. Another difficulty is that the effectiveness of such drugs is often inconsistent and varies from batch to batch.

Genetic engineering makes it possible for these hormones, and other similar protein hormones, to be produced artificially. Cells taken from the ovaries of Chinese hamsters are cultured in huge vats in a kind of soup. Before commencing their active growth, they are modified with the human gene which makes FSH. A fairly similar process is now being used on a research basis to produce LH. The cells then begin to multiply vigorously and massive amounts of hormone can be produced economically and reliably. The method of production allows the active parts of the FSH molecule to be tailored or altered by changing its structure. Thus the genetically engineered drug can be made more or less potent, more or less long-acting.

Genetically engineered FSH may possibly be more potent than its biologically derived equivalents, and the next few years may see a range of more effective preparations of FSH coming into widespread use. Drug companies have been promoting this new generation of drugs very heavily indeed, but so far the only significant improvement has been more freedom from side-effects rather than any serious improvement in pregnancy rates.

The major disadvantage of these drugs is their extra cost. Another is that old-fashioned HMG (derived from biological sources) was a mixture of FSH with a trace of LH. The LH, which is normally merely given immediately before ovulation to trigger the final maturation of the follicle, was regarded as an unwanted contaminant. It was left in the mixture simply because it was too laborious and too expensive to remove. Although it was the FSH which stimulated the follicles to grow, the 'contamination' with LH may have actually been helpful. It turns out that this extra hormone given in tiny amounts may help the ovary to produce better quality eggs.

We shall, unfortunately, have to wait for a genetically engineered LH to add to the rather heavy cocktail we give our patients before we can be sure that we really do have a significant improvement. I remain sceptical that any change in mere drug therapy is going to make a huge difference; probably the big 'breakthrough' will come when we do not need to give these drugs at all.

In vitro maturation of eggs

A much more important advance is under way which may make it possible eventually to dispense with the use of expensive stimulatory drugs altogether. The problem is essentially simple. It is to find a way of maturing eggs outside the body.

To achieve fertilisation the egg has to be properly matured. Immature eggs will not normally fertilise properly, and on the rare occasions they do, they will not produce an embryo. Maturation of the egg is a lengthy process, and takes place over many months (if not years) with a massive spurt during the last menstrual cycle immediately before ovulation. The use of injections of FSH is simply a way of inducing the last spurt artificially, and to get the ovary to produce more mature eggs simultaneously than it would do normally.

The process of maturation is highly complex and is under the control of various genes in the ovary which almost certainly need to be activated in a particular order and in a controlled fashion to produce 'good' eggs. Maturation involves increasing and augmenting the cells immediately surrounding the egg so that it can get its energy requirements. The egg too, as it matures, starts to awaken its own metabolic processes. Maturation changes the unreceptive egg, making it receptive to sperm and capable of penetration. It allows the egg to develop a unique barrier so that normally it can be fertilised by only one sperm. It means placing the chromosomes in order so that they can pair with the chromosomes that come packaged with the sperm to form a new individual with a unique genetic message.

The problem of inducing maturation outside the body artificially, then, is clearly a tall order. But if we could do it, reproductive medicine would undergo a great revolution. Apart from anything else, if we understood the maturation process and its genetic control, we would almost certainly have a method for treating those women who respond poorly to drugs, or who don't ovulate normal eggs when stimulated. But perhaps the most exciting impact is how it would fundamentally change pretty well all infertility treatment.

An adult woman's ovaries contains 400,000 eggs or more. A child has far more. All of these eggs are near the surface of the ovary in a thin layer which is immensely rich in primitive follicles. Normally during a lifetime a few hundred of them are ovulated – in a society like ours between two or three end up as a child. The rest are wasted. One or two square millimetres of ovarian surface tissue – a piece smaller than the head of a match – will contain perhaps 1000 eggs. That is enough eggs for the reproductive lifetime of three women.

If we could take a tiny piece of tissue like that, extract the eggs in the laboratory, store them and mature them *in vitro*, we would truly change fertility treatment and how we think about it. There would be enough eggs for free egg donation if needed. We could treat young women who develop cancers, giving them back their eggs after their radiation or chemotherapy treatments. We could ameliorate the concerns of those women who are reluctant to get pregnant because of a career, allowing egg storage to avoid the ageing process. Many difficult issues will certainly follow.

But one thing is clear. We would make infertility treatment far cheaper, less involved, and much safer. Instead of giving heavy drug treatment to women, we would give a tiny amount of these drugs to the tissue in a glass dish. There would be no ultrasound monitoring and no hormone tests needed for that. No risks of hyperstimulation or discomfort. Eggs matured in the laboratory would simply be matured by the partner's sperm and the embryos replaced in the uterus by a simple procedure of embryo transfer.

So how close are we to all this?

Firstly, it is very easy to take pieces of the ovarian surface. Surgeons doing laparoscopy can do it with no damage or bleeding at all. But it is almost certain that it would not need a laparoscopy. Ovarian tissue could be retrieved just by using a needle, introduced with some local anaesthetic, on an outpatient basis.

Nor is it difficult to store this tissue once it has been retrieved. Dr Outi Hovatta, working in our laboratory on secondment from Finland, has developed simple methods for preserving the ovarian tissue in culture media, and then freezing it in liquid nitrogen. Ovarian tissue treated like this is functional after thawing – Professors Gosden in Leeds and David Baird from Edinburgh have done elegant transplantation experiments in sheep to prove that their fertility can be restored after return of ovarian tissue.

Moreover, it is not too difficult to remove the tiny primordial (primitive) follicles containing the eggs from the ovary. In our laboratory, Dr Ronit Abir managed to do this using careful and delicate dissection. Others have done it by dissolving away the unwanted tissue surrounding the follicles with chemicals.

FSH can be given in tiny amounts to the ovarian follicles in certain culture conditions which allow them to mature, at least to a limited extent. Soon it may be possible to take eggs from those follicles and induce the last stages of the egg maturation process. I suspect that within the next four or five years we may be in a position to attempt to fertilise eggs, treated in this way.

Such an approach will have a radical effect on the availability of IVF. Instead of costing several thousand pounds or dollars (or more) with drugs, an IVF treatment will be easily affordable. It would seem very likely that the whole treatment might cost no more than a few hundred pounds and could be repeated with very little difficulty and minor costs. The convenience for women in terms of the reduction of medicalisation of these treatments is very easy to predict. But much more interesting is the extraordinary control that women will then have over their fertility.

This new technology represents not just an advance in the treatment of infertility. Potentially it has huge social implications for all of society. In future, ovarian storage could become a form of family planning. A woman's declining fertility need no longer be an obstacle to her in mapping out her career. A student could store pieces of ovarian tissue while she was at university studying for her degree, then work hard to establish herself in her chosen career. Then years later when her financial situation was secure and she was in a stable relationship, she could return for her eggs to be fertilised. Even though she may now be in her 40s or even 50s, her eggs would be as fertile as they were when they were first stored twenty years earlier, and becoming pregnant should not present a problem. Biology will always be easier for men, but the gap is closing. Next stop will be the artificial uterus.

Embryo freezing

In an average IVF cycle about nine or ten eggs are collected. About 60 per cent will fertilise but in Britain, in order to limit the risk of multiple births no more than three embryos are transferred to the uterus at the same time. Consequently spare embryos are often left over after many IVF attempts. Embryo freezing offers a couple the opportunity to have their surplus embryos preserved. They can be thawed later for another attempt at getting pregnant later. Frozen embryos can also be donated to other infertile couples. Embryo freezing or cryopreservation, can also be used to preserve the fertilised eggs of women who have malignant diseases such as cancer or leukaemia and who are undergoing treatments with radiation, or chemotherapy with drugs, that may cause sterility.

Freezing of spare embryos for transfer later saves the cost of expensive drugs and much of the cost of a treatment cycle. Transfer of thawed embryos saves expenditure and in most units costs about half to one-third of a full treatment.

To obtain the extremely low temperatures (about minus 200 degrees centigrade) required to keep embryos for long periods, liquid nitrogen is used. The great obstacle to cryopreservation initially was the damage caused to cells when the water within them produced ice-crystals. The solution to this problem has partly been to use 'antifreeze' or cryo-protectants like glycerol. The embryos are bathed in a solution of these cryoprotectants, which gets rid of most of the water in the cells, minimising the degree of ice formation.

The efficiency of embryo freezing has also been improved by the use of specially designed freezing machines. These are programmed by comput-er to freeze tissue or embryos at a precise and usually slow, controlled rate. Programmed freezers are quite expensive. Moreover, before any tissues, eggs, embryos or sperm can be stored using them, a number of carefully established trials have to be done by the embryologists before-hand. Once calibrated, the machine will reproduce the precise rate of freezing and thawing that is required to ensure maximum viability of the particular tissue to be cryopreserved.

The techniques of slow programmed freezing were first worked out in mouse embryos by Dr David Whittingham in the 1970s and 1980s. Embryos from different species require different rates of cooling and thawing, but the principle is basically the same for all embryos. Eggs and sperm, and ovarian and testicular tissue, all require a different recipe to assure the best storage without damage.

Mice embryos have now been kept for 25 years with little deterioration after thawing. David Whittingham conducted a series of simple but elegant experiments whereby, at five-yearly intervals, he removed frozen mouse embryos from liquid nitrogen storage. He then thawed them and then transferred them to the uterus of a recipient mouse. The mouse subsequently gave birth. It turned out that embryos that were frozen for 25 years had the same potential for development as those frozen for five years. Prolonged freezing caused no apparent damage, and it is surmised it would be perfectly possible to keep a frozen embryo for several hundred years without necessarily damaging it in any way.

There is no reason to suppose that freezing human embryos should be any less successful, but I feel slight concern about its complete safety. It is a recognised fact that embryos are less likely to produce a pregnancy after freezing and thawing. Different clinics produce different data, because there is no standard way of reporting the results of embryo freezing, but various results suggest that human embryos after thawing and transfer are only half as likely to produce a baby as those which have been transferred fresh (see page 114). So clearly the freezing process is having some adverse effect.

It is damage which can be clearly seen down a microscope. At the stage when most embryo freezing is done, the embryo is a clump of about four to eight cells. Microscopic inspection after the thawing of what was, for example, an eight-cell embryo before freezing will frequently show that some of its cells are dying, missing or fragmented. Of course, there is the fact that several thousand normal babies have been born after embryo freezing in spite of such damage, and there is no evidence at all of any increase in fetal abnormality. But we do not know what problems may become apparent as these children grow up.

One worry concerns the cryoprotectants which embryo freezing requires. There are various different compounds, of which perhaps the most common is dimethylsulphoxide (DMSO). DMSO is a powerful solvent which can penetrate cell walls very quickly – it is this property which allows it to be used as a carrier to deliver other drugs across the skin. But it is also a potential mutagen, which in high doses has been associated with mutation of the DNA in cells. Because it is such a powerful solvent, it could just possibly dissolve other mutagens within it which went on to cause mutation. Such effects would be likely to go unnoticed for a considerable length of time.

Some experienced embryologists have recorded immediate visible damage to the cell nucleus after freezing and thawing. The nucleus is where the DNA is kept. The DNA is the blue print of the organism, which formulates our inherited characteristics. Some embryologists have reported seeing part of the DNA being excluded from the nucleus of the cell and lying outside it during freezing procedures. This could just possibly be serious. If the DNA was damaged like this, part of the blueprint would be missing.

There is somewhat worrying evidence from the freezing of animal embryos. A group of French scientists, headed by Dr Duliost, examined the long-term effect of freezing embryos in mice. They compared adult mice that had been frozen as embryos with mice which had not been frozen during embryo growth. They reported some unexpected differences in the mice derived from frozen embryos. They tended to grow fatter than usual in old age, and there were some changes in their jaw structure as they grew. Behavioural testing revealed that these mice also displayed different patterns. It is difficult to know what to make of this isolated report. Unfortunately, a number of scientists have written very dismissively of it, but nobody who is critical of it has yet bothered to repeat the work.

One of the problems with freezing is that if it did occasionally cause mutation, the effect would be unlikely to show up in infancy. Mutagenic effects often manifest themselves much later in life, perhaps with a tendency to develop cancers or to be infertile. It was 50 years before we realised that X-rays during pregnancy increased the chance of exposed offspring developing leukaemia in later life.

All this is not to say that embryo freezing causes cancer or infertility, just that it should still be considered more cautiously than it sometimes is. Until the children produced from frozen embryos are fully grown this should be seen as an experimental procedure and we should be cautious about it. At present I personally would only consider embryo freezing when there is no obvious alternative. The following are the main situations when there really is not a realistic alternative:

- For women over 40 years old who cannot afford to wait for another IVF attempt if the first one fails. In this situation it seems reasonable to freeze any spare embryos which can then be thawed and transferred at monthly intervals afterwards.
- For women needing cancer treatment which may make them infertile.
- When a woman becomes ill during IVF. Embryo transfer and pregnancy may make her condition worse. Embryo freezing makes it

possible to preserve her embryos until she is fully recovered, allowing the transfer to be made a few weeks or months later.

- For people receiving a donor embryo. Here a period of quarantine is necessary before the transfer of the embryo to ensure that the donor does not have a serious disease like AIDS.

Egg freezing

Whatever slight doubts there may be about the present safety of cryo-preservation, it is clearly one of the most important advances in IVF technology. Its development as an established procedure will make it possible to overcome many present-day problems. One of the most difficult involves egg donation and the storage of eggs for women having cancer therapy which will produce an early menopause. We have already seen that donor eggs are very difficult to obtain; we find on average only one donor or so for every 50 women wishing to 'adopt' an egg in our clinic (see page 185). If human eggs could be stored in liquid nitrogen, then they could be fertilised later for transfer to women who have no other chance of producing a child. Egg freezing on a big scale would solve the chief objection that using 'spare eggs' from patients undergoing IVF compromises their own treatment. If frozen storage was perfected, then spare eggs could be held until it was clear that the donor's treatment had worked and she had become safely pregnant or even delivered. She could then give approval for her eggs to be fertilised by a recipient woman's husband, without the need to worry about any detrimental effects on her own treatment.

The first baby was born after egg freezing in 1987 by a Dr Chen working in Singapore. The technique used was essentially the same as that which had been established by Alan Trounson's team in Australia, but most workers had pulled away from the idea of egg freezing as animal evidence had shown that there was a potential danger to it. Unlike the copious work using animal embryos, there had been evidence from a limited number of experiments, mostly with mouse eggs, that freezing and thawing might disrupt genetic material in the egg. Dr Peter Braude and Dr Martyn Johnson (now both professors) from Cambridge conducted a number of important experiments which suggested that some offspring could be born with defects whilst at other times these defects were lethal. Dr Chen's work was conducted before proper animal trials had been done. It is, I am afraid, an example of rushing with experimental work in human subjects before proper assessment in animals. Some people may feel that animal research is difficult to accept but reproductive medicine is an excellent example of where it is absolutely essential. I regret to say that Dr Chen's work was not driven out of necessity – it wasn't a last ditch stand to try to save the life of a cancer victim. There were clear safe alternatives for the patients who had these eggs fertilised and transferred. In reproductive medicine we have a special responsibility – not only are the parents our patients, but a child may be produced as a result of what we do. Since Dr Chen's experiments there have been isolated attempts at using frozen/thawed eggs to produce a baby, but egg freezing is still regarded as too risky for clinical use.

Once a reliable method has been perfected, egg freezing will have enormous advantages over embryo freezing. Frozen embryos are a kind of hostage to the fortune of their parents. Should something happen to one or both of them, the disposal of their embryos is always likely to raise legal and ethical difficulties. Unfertilised eggs carry much less moral status, and their disposal would therefore presumably be easier. Egg freezing could, paradoxically, also be safer in the long run. This is because after thawing, a frozen embryo is more or less immediately transferred to the uterus, offering little opportunity to check whether it is growing normally. By contrast, a thawed egg has to be fertilised, which in itself is one test of normality. Thereafter there is the opportunity to observe the subsequent growth of the embryo over several days. If the freeze/thaw process had caused damage, cell division might be disturbed. But most important is the fact that, following Dr Chen's work, a number of different ways of assessing embryo quality are being developed and it will be possible to check whether freezing eggs is actually causing damage to chromosomes or genes.

Zona drilling, assisted hatching and partial zona dissection

Zona drilling was a technique that was first used inadvertently in 1990 at The Hammersmith Hospital. It was used originally as part of a programme to help those couples who carried a genetic disorder in the family. A hole was drilled into the zona pellucida and a cell extracted for analysis.

When we published early results of zona drilling for genetic diagnosis, a number of experts were surprised that the results of our treatment were so good. In spite of the fact that a cell (or even two cells) had been removed from the embryo, the implantation rate after drilling a hole in the zona was higher than the average implantation rate after normal IVF. Consequently, people began to wonder whether zona drilling gave some clinical advantage. It was supposed that by drilling a hole in the zona the outer shell of the egg was weakened and the embryo helped to hatch from the broken egg shell – so-called 'assisted hatching'. In support of this idea was the observation that some eggs (and therefore embryos) were surrounded by a thicker than average zona which was thought to be rather tough. It was presumed that such a tough zona would not readily break spontaneously, as it is supposed to do at around five days after fertilisation. A number of groups started to deliberately drill holes in the zona in women who had poor IVF success rates, or in eggs that they presumed were surrounded by a rather thick zona.

As with so many reproductive techniques, the initial results of assisted hatching were greeted with considerable enthusiasm. However, it was not until 1993 that any controlled trials were done. When they were, it was shown that drilling a hole in the zona seemed to make no difference statistically. However, there was a slight suspicion that women in the older age group did have a slightly better success rate than average when their eggs had a hole drilled in them. The first group to report this was that of Dr Benjamin Fisch in the Beilinson Hospital, in Israel. There is still great doubt as to whether there really is any genuine benefit, but some groups try to drill holes in the zona in the eggs of women over 40. At The Hammersmith we remain unconvinced of any genuine advantage in assisted hatching.

Drilling a hole in the zona can be done by a number of different methods. The egg is held firmly in a suction pipette made of glass, a pipette which is similar to that used during immobilisation of the egg for ICSI. A tiny drop of acid can be introduced on the outside of the egg, and this will burn a small hole removing about five per cent of the zona. Alternatively, a nick can be made in the zona with a very fine piece of glass, delivered by a micro manipulator. This – so-called partial zona dissection (PZD) – is simply another way of opening up the zona by making a slightly larger injury in the zona than is achieved by drilling. It appears to have no specific advantages over other methods. A third technique is to use a laser beam to drill one or more holes in the zona.

In Britain, the HFEA will not allow zona drilling unless the unit has a specific licence for it. The HFEA remains unconvinced of its value, and is concerned that it could possibly cause damage. In particular, creating a hole in the zona could allow micro-organisms such as viruses to enter the embryo and in consequence it is just faintly possible that abnormalities of the embryos could develop. In my view, however, zona drilling is both harmless and useless. It does have the disadvantage to patients that units that employ it often charge considerable sums of money to execute the procedure.

Embryo selection

Because of the low chance of any single embryo successfully implanting and resulting in pregnancy, IVF clinics try to transfer more than one embryo simultaneously. This brings with it an increased risk of miscarriage and multiple birth. Since the advent of IVF, the incidence of multiple birth in Britain has more than doubled. Most triplets, and nearly all quadruplets, that are born have been conceived following assisted reproductive treatments of one kind or another; about half of the total come as a result of IVF. High-order multiple birth usually spells disaster. Triplets virtually never go to term; if they survive pregnancy at all, most are born six to eight weeks prematurely. Having three or four babies develop in the womb simultaneously greatly increases the hazards of pregnancy. High blood pressure, toxaemia, diabetes and blood clots are all much more likely. Delivery by Caesarean section is nearly always needed and most of these very premature babies will require intensive nursing, sometimes for several weeks, in incubators.

The cost to the National Health Service is enormous, and clearly a major breakthrough in IVF will be the ability to transfer a single embryo without severely compromising the treatment's rate of success. Researchers have devised a number of tests on embryos in culture to ascertain which are most likely to be viable to implant.

One of the most promising of these tests involves the non-invasive assessment of an embryo's metabolism. The assumption is that the more energy an embryo is using, the more likely it is to be growing actively and therefore to be viable. Hours after fertilisation the embryo is placed in a tiny droplet of fluid so small that it can scarcely be seen with the naked eye. The droplet together with the embryo in it are placed under a special silicone oil which isolates it from the atmosphere. The medium in which the embryo is allowed to grow contains a measured amount of carbohydrate. After 24 hours the embryo can be removed from its droplet and placed in a new freshly prepared one. The original droplet can then be analysed to see how much of the original carbohydrate has been consumed by the embryo.

Measurements of several hundred embryos have consistently shown that the more viable embryos consume more carbohydrate and are more metabolically active. One interesting finding is that male embryos are, on average, eighteen per cent more active than female embryos. Men, it seems, are more aggressive from the moment of conception. But energy consumption is not reliable as a discriminatory test. There is so much variation in metabolic activity from embryo to embryo, irrespective of sex, that the test cannot determine viability in any single instance. Carbohydrate metabolism is a very basic process, and even cells which are about to die may consume considerable amounts of it.

It is likely that in the near future other forms of metabolic measurement will provide a much more accurate test of an embryo's viability. One promising area of research is to look at what amino acids are taken up by the embryo. By measuring the depletion of amino acids from culture media over a fixed period of time, an individual embryo's growth potential can be gauged.

It may also be possible to measure the various growth factors that the cells in the embryo need to divide. Growth factors are chemical messengers which attach themselves to receptors on the cell wall. Attachment to receptors leads to the generation of further messages within the cell which tell it to grow and divide. It is already known that embryos require growth factors of various sorts to stimulate their growth and researchers are assessing which growth factors are most important, and which may be needed to provide the best culture environment. The embryo itself may produce different growth factors as its own genes are switched on. These growth factors are messengers which tell the lining cells of the uterine cavity that the embryo is present. It is likely that these messages are important in preparing the endometrium for implantation.

Better culture

Embryos of different species require different chemicals to achieve their best growth. Human embryo culture media have always contained glucose, because it seemed obvious that this substance, the basic energy-giving substance for all mammals, would be ideal. But it has recently been discovered that even quite small amounts of glucose may reduce or prevent growth in mice embryos in the first two days after fertilisation. It seems that in the first 48 hours of development, the genes which control our energy requirements are promoting an anaerobic system. Glucose is only used for aerobic metabolism, and aerobic metabolism does not start until two or three days after fertilisation. A surfeit of glucose in the early stages of life may therefore be a bad thing.

There is little convincing evidence that glucose is similarly harmful to early human IVF embryos. However it does seem that they may develop a bit better when other energy sources are available to them. Certainly it is clear that the culture media currently used are probably far from ideal. There are several pieces of important evidence.

As far as we can tell, human embryos obtained by IVF grow more slowly than after natural fertilisation and incubation in the fallopian tube. It is difficult to be sure because it is extraordinarily difficult to get access to naturally fertilised human eggs. Some very elegant work by Professor Horacio Croxatto in Chile, in the Catholic University of Santiago, gives a clue as to how quickly the human blastocyst stage is reached. When he flushed embryos from the fallopian tube and uterus undergoing sterilisation (remarkably bold for a Professor in a Catholic university) he found that they were about one day further advanced in development than we see in modern IVF media. Blastocysts had formed in the uterine cavity within 96 to 110 hours after ovulation – around four days after ovulation, rather than the five days after ovulation we see in IVF.

In most IVF units any single embryo transferred to the uterus on the second day after fertilisation has about a ten to fifteen per cent chance of becoming a baby. In some units, where extra care is taken over laboratory techniques, the chance can rise to a maximum of around 20–25 per cent. This variation in the success rates is further evidence that the artificial conditions in which embryos are kept in culture laboratories are crucial.

Human embryos also have a reduced chance of survival if grown for more than three days in culture media outside the body. Even in the best laboratories, the best chance of a four or five day old embryo grown *in vitro* implanting after transfer is around 40 per cent (see also blastocyst culture below). Most attempts to achieve pregnancy after transfer have been less successful. By comparison, the work of Dr Buster in California in 1985 was interesting. He collected naturally fertilised human blastocysts from women by uterine flushing. He then transferred them to the uterus of women who wanted to adopt an embryo. The pregnancy rate was 60 per cent. Similar results were obtained by Dr Formigli, in Italy, some years later. All this rather suggests that the body provides a better environment.

Dr Kate Hardy, at The Hammersmith Hospital, has shown that human IVF embryos, at an equivalent stage in their development usually have fewer cells in them than embryos which have grown naturally inside the body. Her studies also show a large number of defects in human IVF embryos. Dying cells are very common, and the proteins which control the messages between one cell and the next – the gap junctions – are often deranged. She has found that many embryos also have abnormalities of their nuclei, and there are also more chromosomal abnormalities than one might perhaps expect. Of course, some of these abnormalities may be due to fertilisation of abnormal eggs – possibly the massive doses of stimulatory drugs that we give to induce ovulation may be deleterious. But it is very likely that many of these abnormalities are in part due to inefficiencies in the culture system.

Several experiments with culture media are being conducted. It is now clear that the correct concentration of carbohydrate may promote embryonic development and the wrong concentration inhibit it. We still do not know what the ideal level is for the human embryo, but it is likely that its requirements change during development. It seems that the carbohydrate, pyruvate, is needed for the first two days, but after that glucose is needed. It may well be that the culture media needs to be changed according to the precise stage of the embryo's development.

Research is also being conducted into the embryo's need for amino acids, the building blocks from which our various proteins are made. There are twenty common different amino acids. Perhaps one of the most neglected in embryo cultures is glutamine, which some embryos seem to need for best growth. This requirement varies not merely between different animal species but even between different strains of the same species. Most mouse embryos for example need it, although there are some strains of laboratory mice whose embryos can develop normally in media which contain no glutamine at all. Our recent research with human embryos suggests that the presence of glutamine in the culture media may enormously enhance growth in the early stages. Once research has determined the correct proportion in which it should be used, then its addition may greatly improve current culture media. There are also a whole range of other compounds, including inorganic metals and various salts, which need to be tested and could make a considerable difference to the success of IVF.

The most exciting prospect is probably the study of growth factors. Dr Antony Lighten, one of our PhD students, has been working on one group of growth factors – those which are similar in chemical structure to insulin. In the adult, the action of insulin is very well known – it is responsible for controlling sugar metabolism and without it an individual develops diabetes. In early embryos, insulin plays a very different role. It acts on other substances within the embryonic cells and gives instruction for growth. Dr Lighten has studied two molecules very much like insulin. The first is insulin-like growth factor 1 (IGF-1), the second is insulin-like growth factor 2 (IGF-2). Both of these stimulate growth and cell division in early embryonic development. Antony Lighten has examined the genes responsible for the production of these compounds, and determined when they are switched on during development.

Dr Lighten's work shows that the human embryo has chemical receptors for IGF-1 and IGF-2, and is capable of producing IGF-2 on its own. In producing its own IGF-2, the embryo in a way carries the seeds of its own success. But IGF-1 is not being produced. That substance is in the fallopian tube in large amounts, and in the uterus. It is not present in the normal media which all laboratories use for embryo cultures. The thought occurred to us that perhaps its addition would help embryonic growth. It turns out that when it is added to the medium containing a dividing embryo, its chance of survival almost doubles, and the number of cells it contains improves markedly. There can be no doubt that this is the effect of the added growth factors, because if the receptors of IGF-1 are deliberately blocked by giving an antibody, and then IGF is added, no extra growth occurs.

We have not yet added these substances to the culture of embryos that are to be transferred. One would hope that pregnancy rates might well improve. But to tamper with an embryo that is to be transferred requires careful thought. We do not know the ideal dose of growth factor. What might happen if we gave too much, for example? Could this cause abnormalities? Before such an experiment is done – even though so many desperate human patients are prepared to try anything – careful thought is required, more measurement needed and then appropriate approaches made to the ethical committees.

This work has been made possible and facilitated by examining the genes which control early development. This basic method is, I think, important. Even if insulin-like growth factors themselves do not turn out to be the elixir of life, then certainly we shall find other compounds, currently missing in media, which will change IVF. Looking at what the embryonic genes express is a clear indication of what they most need for survival.

Blastocyst culture

At present, embryos are almost always transferred on the second or third day after fertilisation. This is not the time when an embryo would normally be present in the uterus after a natural conception. At that stage of development, it would normally be in the fallopian tube, where the environment is different. It has long been thought that the environment in the uterus is not ideal for an embryo which is less than three days old. Indeed before the first embryo transfers were done, there was always the suggestion that the fluid in the uterus might even be toxic to early embryos. Moreover, at the time of the second or third day after fertilisation, the lining of the uterus, the endometrium, may be out of synchrony. By this I mean that the embryo, in culture, possibly grows at a slower rate than it would in its natural place, the fallopian tube. Meantime the rate of growth of the endometrium is possibly accelerated, or at least changed, because of the stimulation caused by extra oestrogen resulting from ovarian stimulation. It is a very complex equilibrium and is not fully understood. Theoretically, the ideal time to transfer an embryo to the uterus would be when it is ready to implant it and, of course, at the time when the endometrium is most receptive to implantation. This should be sometime after the blastocyst is naturally formed, at least five or six days after fertilisation.

Unfortunately, at the present time IVF culture systems are simply not efficient enough to provide the ideal environment for blastocyst development. When attempts to grow blastocysts *in vitro* are made, fewer than 30 per cent or 40 per cent of embryos survive to that stage. Moreover, their growth in culture is retarded and, after five days, many of them have half the normal number of cells. There is therefore doubt about their potential for further development. Theoretically, although a 50 to 60 per cent pregnancy rate might be expected after transfer of a single blastocyst, no unit has remotely achieved this. The table following gives the results seen from various units. The best come just close to this ideal but remember that in all these units most of the embryos did not become blastocysts. There is a high attrition rate and the implantation rate per fertilised egg is no better, and probably worse, than the best results achieved with the transfer of embryos on day two or day three after fertilisation. Moreover, the results in the table were generally obtained in optimal circumstances, mostly in young, selected patients, and when everything was in favour of a pregnancy being established.

Research worker	Co-culture	Transfers	Pregnancy %	Implantation per embryo %
Menezo et al. (1983)	yes	172	42	25
Bolton et al. (1991)	no	29	10	7
Olivennes et al. (1994)	yes	104	34	18
*Forsdahl et al. (1994)	no	27	48	39
Scholtes et al. (1996)	no	410	25	12
Scholtes et al. (1998)	no	946	34	12 to 23
Scholtes et al. (1998)	no	586	8	6
*Gardner et al. (1998)	no	8	63	46
Gardner et al. (1998)	no	15	47	21

*Note that high implantation rate was only achieved in two small series

But it is clearly worth persisting with research. One of the great advantages of blastocyst culture might be that, with transfer of a single normal blastocyst we could reduce the incidence of multiple pregnancy. If we were able to get a 50 to 60 per cent pregnancy rate with the transfer of just one blastocyst, there would be no justifiable indication for transferring more than two embryos. Indeed, the ideal would be to transfer single embryos in repeated cycles, until a pregnancy occurred.

If it could be made more efficient, blastocyst transfer would allow better selection of healthy embryos. By keeping embryos in culture for longer periods of time, those that have no potential for development and are bound to die before implantation, could be 'weeded out'. Assessment of the chemicals that embryos were producing might also improve information about their health. The minute differences in metabolic activity on the second and third day that we observed in our laboratories are too slight to make a diagnosis between a normal or abnormal embryo with any certainty. By the fifth or sixth day when there are far more cells in the embryo, it is likely that such measurements would lead to more meaningful results. An embryo clearly using more energy might well be more likely to implant. Culture to the blastocysts stage would have other possible advantages. As a healthy blastocyst should contain more than 100 cells, analysis of DNA for preimplantation genetic diagnosis could, if needed, be done more reliably. There would be the possibility of removing more than just one or two cells for assessment.

There remain many problems with blastocyst culture. We do not yet know the ideal environment for embryos at that stage. A number of scientists have mapped out constituents for the media, and one possible way of improving blastocyst development is to change the media repeatedly during five days of development. With each change, new constituents which are needed for the next stage of growth, may be added. For example, at the beginning of culture, glucose might be omitted from the medium. Later on, it might be added and, as development progresses, different growth factors might be added to the media as well as different amino acids. All this cookery would depend on what the embryo was found to need at each stage of development.

Some researchers have tried a system of co-culture, that is growing embryos in the presence of other cells. When embryos are grown in co-culture with cells taken from other tissues, they may act as 'helpers'. For example, helper cells taken from a fallopian tube may produce growth factors such as IGF-1 (see page 133). However, although early results showed considerable promise, experiments in this direction have recently been rather disappointing. Co-culture is a good idea but may not be valuable. Moreover there is the concern that it is difficult to find suitable donated cells from humans. Any donated cell may carry with it some unexpected virus and for this reason, such systems may be hard to develop.

I have no doubt that it will be possible eventually to grow human blastocysts in culture reliably. It is largely a matter of understanding the physiology involved. Once the problem is solved, IVF will become much easier, embryo transfer will have far better success rates and the risk of multiple pregnancy will become progressively less.

Implantation

There has been a huge increase in the understanding of embryonic development over the last twenty years. We now have a better idea of what is a normal or an abnormal embryo. But the ideal circumstances and environment for that embryo to implant remain mysterious. We know remarkably little about endometrial development. This has been a rather neglected field which only now is starting to be studied. We are going to learn a great deal about which genes produce the proteins which are needed for implantation. We shall soon understand more too about the chemical messages the embryo gives out by which it signals its presence in the cavity of the uterus. These signals require a response from the uterine lining and probably initiate the cascade of events which follow, and which dictate human survival in the womb.

A number of interesting genes in the uterine lining are now being studied. One laboratory that has made great progress in this field is that headed by Professor Steve Smith, at Cambridge University. Some of these important genes may not be functioning properly in some women and may therefore be a cause of IVF failure. They may also, of course, cause 'unexplained' infertility. These genes, and the proteins they produce, can sometimes be identified using advanced laboratory techniques and by microscope study after special methods of staining. Unfortunately, there is no established test that can be used yet during a 'live' treatment cycle so there is no practical benefit, but this lack is likely to change within three to five years.

One research approach has been to look at pieces of uterine lining taken during treatment cycles, and during cycles when women have been treated with hormones to mimic a pregnancy cycle. Using the powerful electron microscope, it is possible to see changes on the surface of the endometrium which are thought to signal its most receptive time. At this time when it is ready for implantation, the endometrium forms little blisters, called pinopodes, on its surface. These blisters are probably secretions which may contain molecules which help the endometrium and embryo stick to each other, initiating the first stage of implantation.

We now have the feeling that some women do not have normal development of these blisters. Their absence may be a cause of failure of implantation and further study of how they are formed, what they contain, and how long they stay is likely to be fruitful.

Antibodies preventing implantation

There has been a great deal of recent interest in the antibodies which may affect the way the pregnancy implants or how an early pregnancy takes. One is the anticardiolipin antibody; another is the lupus anticoagulant which is present in some diseases which change our immune status. Both these are found to be raised in many women who are completely disease-free, but are prone to recurrent miscarriage. One treatment is to give these women daily doses of aspirin if they are miscarrying repeatedly. There is statistical evidence that this seems to work. Another treatment, which is much more risky, is to give an anticoagulant called heparin. Heparin thins the blood, prevents clotting and of course may thus promote unwanted bleeding. There is also less evidence that heparin is of real value for repeated miscarriage. In some places, the USA for example, some of these patients are also given corticosteroids, usually in the form of prednisolone. Steroids, too, are not without risk and one cannot but feel that this 'polypharmacy' is bad medicine, born out of desperation and frustration.

Because these medicines have been tried with equivocal results in recurrent miscarriage, it seemed logical to some people to try them after repeated failure of embryo transfer, even when these antibodies are not present. There is a kind of ill-thought out notion that these unfortunate women may be losing a very early implantation. Not surprisingly, the American vogue has hit some private clinics in Britain. There is absolutely no evidence that heparin or steroids work, but they certainly may cause complications, including bleeding and gastric ulceration.

In my view the giving of these drugs, including aspirin, is only justified when there is clear evidence that these antibodies are present in abnormal amounts in the blood stream. Even then, they are of very dubious value. Our own view is that aspirin may be of benefit and we are currently conducting a trial using it, in collaboration with Professor Lesley Regan at St Mary's Hospital, London. Aspirin is at least relatively harmless, so a trial of this kind has no serious ethical problems.

8

Legislation and the role of the HFEA

The introduction of IVF with the birth of Louise Brown in 1978 caused an ethical and biological revolution. Humans now had access to their very genesis and it caused a wave which still impacts on our understanding of ourselves. Britain led the way in developing *in vitro* fertilisation, with Australia and the USA not far behind. Nevertheless, it was a comparatively long time before any legal restraints were placed either on the practice of IVF, or the research on embryos which led to its development.

The Warnock Commission

In Britain, a Royal Commission was set up under the chairmanship of Dame Mary Warnock (now Baroness Warnock), and this reported to the British Government in July 1984. A somewhat similar process took place in Australia. Following The Human Embryo Experimentation Bill (1985), a Senate Select Committee chaired by Senator Michael Tate from Tasmania considered the issues raised by embryo research and freezing of human embryos. In the United States, there was less unified national action, largely because individual states are empowered to legislate individually on such issues. Nonetheless, the federal government was concerned about the problems raised by research on human embryos and it decided that it would not fund any such scientific endeavour.

In Britain, the Government was reluctant to introduce legislation too hastily. The Warnock Commission had given a broadly permissive view on embryo experimentation. It agreed that such research was of substantial benefit. After two years of taking evidence, it had found that until the development of the primitive streak – the first signs of organ formation about two weeks after fertilisation – the human embryo was not clearly established. The Commission recognised that most human embryos did not survive beyond this stage of development. Because of this, and because twinning commonly occurs during the first fourteen days of life, the Commission agreed unanimously that such early embryos could hardly be regarded as 'individuals'.

The main recommendations of the Warnock Commission were:

1. The establishment of a licensing authority to regulate research and infertility treatments, with an arrangement for licensing practitioners and researchers.
2. No embryo used for research should be transferred to the uterus.
3. Trans-species fertilisation should be a criminal offence.
4. Human embryos should not be placed in the uterus of another species.
5. There should be no right of ownership over the human embryo.
6. Egg and sperm donation, as well as embryo donation, should be permitted with appropriate controls.
7. No human embryo should be kept in culture beyond fourteen days.
8. The consent of the couple involved should be sought for any research on, or disposal of, embryos. There should be written consent for all acts involving donor insemination.
9. There should be follow-up studies of children born as a result of the new reproductive techniques.
10. Sale and purchase of eggs, sperm and embryos should be permitted under conditions prescribed by the licensing authority.
11. Donation of eggs and sperm should be anonymous.
12. Semen donors should have no legal rites or duties in relation to their genetic children conceived as a result of donation.
13. Counselling should be available for all those undergoing treatment.
14. Children should have access to basic information regarded their genetic origin on reaching the age of eighteen.
15. Embryos should be allowed to be stored frozen for up to ten years.
16. Specialist infertility clinics should be established within the NHS, separate from routine gynaecological clinics, and there should be NHS funding for IVF.
17. A higher priority should be given to infertility treatments.
18. Surrogacy arrangements should effectively be banned.

The recommendations of the Warnock Commission were not unanimous. Two out of the sixteen members felt that surrogacy should be permitted at least for the time being. They wanted concrete evidence that it really was harmful. Three other members recommended that all embryo experimentation should be banned on the grounds that it was tampering with the beginnings of human life, which should be sacrosanct.

Parliamentary activity

There were rather ill-informed, emotional debates in both Houses of Parliament after Warnock reported but the British Government showed little interest in implementing any of these recommendations. Other governments also showed interest in Warnock, but tended to drag their feet over deciding about these difficult and contentious issues. I suppose that it was inevitable that 'right to life' groups around the world were incensed that governments were slow to legislate to limit or prevent embryo experimentation. In addition, the Catholic Church was particularly vociferous because it viewed the fertilised egg as the beginning of human life, after which time the embryo should, in its opinion, be sacrosanct. Any interference with human embryos was seen as being essentially similar to abortion.

In Britain, pressure was building and Members of Parliament were being increasingly lobbied to introduce restrictive law. Most pressure came from the organisations Life and The Society for the Protection of the Unborn Child. At the beginning of 1985, angered by the slow and careful deliberations of the Warnock Commission and the reluctance of government to legislate, individual MPs were invited to introduce legislation. They found a champion in Enoch Powell who introduced a private member's bill 'The Unborn Child (Protection) Bill' at the end of 1984. It is of interest that in Australia, a similar restrictive proposal was introduced in April 1985 by Senator Brian Harradine 'An Act to prohibit experiments involving the use of human embryos created by *in vitro* fertilisation'. In both cases, these Members of Parliament attempted to prohibit any experiment which was not of any 'therapeutic benefit to the embryo'. Were such Bills to become law, it would be permissible to conduct embryo research but only providing the embryo was returned to its mother's uterus after the experiment. Enoch Powell, in attempting to introduce such legislation, was effectively condoning what he regarded as a human subject being used as a guinea pig. Quite characteristically, with the conviction that he was absolutely infallible, Mr Powell never even bothered to visit a department where embryo research was being conducted, nor for that matter visit an infertility clinic and talk to the patients there.

The Bill had many iniquitous provisions. Apart from exhibiting a failure to understand the enormity of the issues surrounding the transfer of an embryo to the uterus after experimentation, it directly attacked IVF treatment. It stipulated that all women having IVF should seek prior permission in writing from the Secretary of State. This was clearly an infringement of personal liberty unparalleled in medical history. Fortunately, Powell's Bill did not become law. Had it done so, it is possible that other countries might have followed a British example and progress in reproductive research, which has importance far beyond the treatment of fertility disorders, would have been severely curtailed. Such was the ignorance of most Members of Parliament of the time, that it could easily have done so and at the time there was much international scrutiny of what the British Parliament was doing about these complex issues. There was, in 1985, a substantial majority of MPs in favour of banning embryo research and the 'right-to-life' caucus were well organised and orchestrated.

At Second Reading in the House of Commons, Powell had an overwhelming vote. A majority of 172 votes – nearly two-thirds – was in favour of banning all research on embryos. Fortunately, being a Private Member's Bill, the Committee stages were rather delayed, and the Bill was eventually 'talked out' by a series of procedural methods. I remember all this very vividly, as I sat up night after night writing briefing notes to sympathetic MPs in an attempt at delaying the passage. On one occasion, after an all-night sitting of the Committee, I worked writing briefs in tandem with Dr Ann MacLaren, one of the most distinguished embryologists of our time. We managed to collate just enough material for our friendly MPs so that the Committee ran out of time just after what should have been breakfast – with five minutes less written material, the Committee stages would have been completed and Powell's Bill might have become law.

Over the next three or four years, there was a series of attempts to introduce severely restrictive legislation by different private Members of Parliament. Without Government support they had very little chance of success, but each motion they tabled caused a flurry of nervous activity from our side. By 1989 it became clear that the Government was to produce its own Bill, to be launched in the House of Lords. Since the Powell Bill, however, there had been a significant change of public opinion. There had been intense and prolonged public debate about the status of the human embryo, with an inevitable amount of detailed media coverage. In addition, publicity given to IVF meant that infertility, and the severe distress it commonly caused so many couples, was increasingly in the news. Both the public and MPs could see the logical connection between headlines and photographs of happily pregnant women and the need to protect the research which had clearly promoted healthy family life.

Voluntary regulation

Powell and his Bill had one very useful effect on IVF. His virulent attacks on IVF and the integrity of the doctors and scientists involved with it, united the professionals. Within weeks of the failure of his 'Unborn Children (Protection) Bill', the Medical Research Council and the Royal College of Obstetricians and Gynaecologists had started procedures which led to voluntary regulation of IVF, along the lines that Warnock had proposed. Without exception, this was welcomed by physicians and scientists. Indeed, these two professions had been instrumental in stimulating these bodies into being active.

A regulatory body, the Voluntary Licensing Authority (VLA) was set up under the excellent, wise chairmanship of Dame Mary Donaldson. Without exception, all IVF clinics, both private and public submitted to inspections by its team of clinicians, scientists and lay people. It ran on lines very much like those of the Government's own body which was set up later in 1991. It was, however, rather more flexible in much of its approach. The VLA awarded licences and assured reasonable clinical standards; it confirmed that donor sperm and eggs were being used along lines suggested by Warnock; above all, it made certain that research was being conducted on proper ethical principles and conformed to standards which the Warnock Committee had recommended. The VLA also produced statistics regarding national success rates after IVF and some of the complications of treatment. These activities were funded by the two official bodies which initiated it. Once it was clear by 1989, that the Government was to introduce legislation, the VLA renamed itself the Interim Licensing Authority or ILA. Throughout the existence of both the VLA and later the ILA, there was only one case of a doctor or scientist refusing to accept the guidelines and recommendations of the voluntary regulators. This concerned the question regarding the number of embryos which could safely be transferred to the uterus – after some dissent, this one doctor agreed to abide by the ruling of the regulators.

The Human Fertilisation and Embryology Act

All this activity by the profession, together with improved public understanding, meant that, in Britain, the climate for the new reproductive technologies was much more receptive. When the Government's own Bill, The Human Fertilisation and Embryology Bill, was introduced into the

House of Lords in 1990, it won an unopposed Second Reading. It was introduced by The Lord Chancellor, Lord MacKay of Clashfern, in a typically elegant and beautifully worded speech. It was a most helpful contribution to the understanding of the whole field. Most peers were strongly supportive of the new technology. There was suspicion from some of the hereditary peers about the use of donor eggs and sperm – the peers in the House by accident of birth seemed more concerned about primogeniture than most of the rest of their Lordships. Some of the speeches opposing the technology when reread some nine years later now seem remarkably cranky, unreasonably suspicious and containing antique argument. For the most part, the atmosphere showed the House of Lords at its best. The argument was strongly favourable with an intelligent balance between the benefits of IVF and the real ethical risks. Once the Bill reached the Commons, it was equally clear that there had been a major change in public opinion. The debate was totally different in character from that five years earlier. There was widespread approval for IVF and the use of donor sperm, and an overwhelming majority – a vote of 173 – entered the division lobby in favour of controlled, regulated research on human embryos. Ironically, this was almost the identical majority (but reversed) that Powell had achieved five years earlier. The Bill passed into law amidst amazing scenes of rejoicing on the floor of the Commons.

The establishment of the HFEA

In broad terms, the Human Fertilisation and Embryology Act (1990) followed the Warnock recommendations very closely indeed. The regulatory authority, The Human Fertilisation and Embryology Authority (HFEA) which was set up, commenced work in 1991. Its main remit was as follows:

1. To grant appropriate licences to clinical or research centres for the storage of human gametes (eggs or sperm) or embryos.
2. To regulate research involving human embryos by operating a licence system to centres.
3. To grant licences to centres offering any treatments involving donated gametes or embryos.
4. To licence any centre wishing to conduct treatments involving the creation of a human embryo outside the body (IVF).
5. To maintain a central register of all treatments given involving donated gametes or embryos, or treatments involving IVF.
6. To publish the services which the Authority provides and which treatment centres provide.

7. To give advice and information to licensed centres where appropriate.
8. To publish a Code of Practice giving guidance to centres on how they should carry out licensed activities.
9. To give advice to donors and prospective donors, to people seeking treatment or storage, or people considering whether to do so.

One bone of contention was the issue of who should pay for all this regulation. Parliament had capped the budget of the HFEA and had only offered a relatively modest sum; consequently the HFEA was empowered to charge a licence fee – separate fees being charged for a licence to conduct clinical treatment, and for each registered research project. In addition, each individual IVF treatment or donor insemination (DI) treatment had the imposition of a 'tax': £30 for IVF and £7 for a DI cycle. One has the very strong feeling that, ever since it was established, the HFEA has been chronically short of money.

The membership of the HFEA

The first Chairman of the HFEA was a lawyer, with twenty other members. All were appointed by the Secretary of State for Health. There were five doctors, three scientists involved with reproductive biology, one nurse and eleven lay members. This last group included a well-known actress, a senior official from the Bank of England, a Bishop, and a television executive, all representing the interests of the wider community. Key individuals within the HFEA were the executive group and I would like to pay tribute to the excellent work of the first Chief Executive, Flora Goldhill, and her Deputy, Hugh Whittall, who did a great deal to ensure smooth relationships between the regulators and the regulated – no mean task.

Although it was there to regulate and impose proper legal restrictions on clinics and their research, it was widely welcomed by doctors and scientists with a broad consensus of approval and the wish to co-operate. The HFEA initially had the great advantage that there was this broad agreement amongst the professionals. Indeed, they had a sense of relief that this important treatment could continue. There was also a feeling of pride amongst most people working in the field of research and clinical IVF that Britain had taken an international lead and was showing the world the way forward.

It was also true that, at the time, at least some members of the HFEA recognised that professionals, who are deeply knowledgeable about their own field, could only be 'ruled' with their agreement and consensus.

Without this tacit support of any body of this kind, there is always the concern that individuals who are regulated will find their way around regulations.

The issue of patient, and donor, confidentiality

There were several important issues facing the new Authority when it was established in 1991. The first was the issue of patient confidentiality. Unfortunately, the original Act of Parliament had been written too tightly. Section 33(5) prevented any person licensed to provide treatment from giving any information about a patient to another person who was unlicensed. This meant that IVF doctors were not able to give routine but important medical details to a patient's general practitioner – even in cases of emergency. The ridiculous consequences were potentially dangerous. For example it meant that, should an IVF patient become ill or collapse following the administration of any drug given in an IVF clinic, that clinic could not respond effectively to an urgent phone call by the troubled GP who might be trying to find out what was happening to his ill patient. This could be potentially disastrous for the very person the law was trying to protect. It also meant that IVF patients' records could not be kept in the filing system of a hospital, because unlicensed practitioners, nurses and records clerks would have access to confidential information – even if the patient's own consent for access had been given. Oddly the law also meant that, in the case of a legal claim against a doctor by a patient, a doctor could not defend himself in a proper court of law or in front of the General Medical Council – as to do so would be breaking the patient's confidentiality. This issue was eventually resolved after the intervention of the Secretary of State, but Parliament had to rush through a special amendment to the original Act in 1992 to avoid this ludicrous problem. In my view, even now the law is too tight. I fail to understand why one particular kind of reproductive treatment should be so much more private than say surgery on the fallopian tube, termination of pregnancy, or indeed a heart bypass operation. It implies a stigma about IVF that I find uncomfortable.

The Act of Parliament required a register to be kept of patients and information regarding donors of gametes. Consequently, a second issue with which the HFEA was faced was the problem of what to do about sperm that had been in storage from before the Act of 1990 came into force. Before 1990 the name of any donor did not have to go on record, but the Act of Parliament required a confidential record of the identity of the donor to be kept. Before these regulations, the details concerning the donor were not always recorded; moreover, in some circumstances the new requirements for screening for viral and bacteriological diseases, and the period of quarantine had not been implemented. In addition, in some cases, there were embryos in frozen storage that had been derived from donated sperm where the genetic parentage was not on record. The Authority ruled that it would amend its requirement for information so that for a limited time such sperm could be used. Rather than direct the destruction of existing embryos, it also ruled that these might be used to produce a pregnancy. Some parents had already had a child from a particular anonymous donor and wanted to have a sibling from the same genetic father. The HFEA also waived its restriction in these circumstances providing there was a written request from the woman concerned – note that, oddly, the prospective father played no part in the HFEA's thinking. In each of the circumstances just described, the registration of the donor's name could be omitted only if it was not known to the centre, or the donor had refused consent to allow it to be recorded.

Licensing the centres

The main activity of the new Authority was licensing centres. After its first meeting the HFEA listed its objectives in licensing:

1. To ensure that no prohibited activities take place and that no activities for which a licence is required are undertaken except under licence.
2. To secure public confidence and the confidence of centres that the Authority is maintaining a fair and consistent framework for licensing.
3. To assure the public and Parliament that the research work which is undertaken under licence is necessary and within the conditions set out in the Act.
4. To assure the public that centres operate to certain minimum standards.

To make this activity possible, it was necessary to arrange for inspection teams to visit each licensed centre, and to visit each centre applying for a new licence. In this respect the HFEA followed the basic procedure which had been adopted by the VLA before the Act of Parliament. The HFEA set up an inspectorate; approximately 60 or so professionals were invited to become inspectors. Typically, an inspection team might comprise four people: a clinician, a scientist, a lay member – for example a nurse, counsellor, or social worker – and a member of the HFEA. Most of the clinicians and scientists were themselves involved in IVF, and of course as they were practising in Britain, were subject to the licensing system themselves.

This, to my mind, created the first beginnings of a potentially serious conflict within the regulatory framework. How could the gamekeepers keep a completely impartial mind when they themselves were, under other circumstances, poachers? It has also to be born in mind that IVF has always had a strong commercial flavour. Simply put, the NHS was not supporting much IVF at all, and consequently the great majority of patients had to go for treatment on a fully private basis. This trend, already significant in 1991, has become much more serious in recent years, particularly with reforms in the funding of the NHS. Most IVF clinics required sufficient income to be viable, and by 1991, there was already increasing competition between clinics. On the academic side, too, there was considerable competition – particularly competition to get research grants and similar support. Moreover, IVF was seen by the media as a 'glamorous' area of medicine and there was worrying evidence of clinics, even those based in academic establishments, trying to attract media attention to the 'latest breakthrough'. Empowering competing professionals to be part of the licensing (rather than regulatory) process was not particularly sound. Certainly, it would hardly seem to fulfil the criterion (2) above 'To secure public confidence and the confidence of centres that the Authority is maintaining a fair and consistent framework for licensing'.

The composition of the inspectorate was no great cause for concern initially. Out of the 60 appointees, only some fifteen were involved in IVF. Nevertheless, there is clear evidence that inspections were inconsistent from the inception of the HFEA. I know for certain that, early on, my own unit had very friendly inspections while neighbouring colleagues had a much tougher time over comparable issues. This problem has become progressively worse as more and more inspectors are needed, and as inevitably they have been increasingly recruited from the IVF clinics. I have absolute confidence that the HFEA has tried hard to maintain uniformity in the inspection procedures. A shopping list of questions is drawn up and there is a standard framework for every inspection.

Nevertheless, my experience in my own unit at The Hammersmith Hospital has varied greatly over the years since the HFEA has been inspecting it. The inspectors with whom I have been personally friendly have always been much more tolerant. Sometimes, the inconsistency has been bizarre. As part of an inspection, the inspecting team examines any patient information literature and vets it, presumably to make sure it is of proper quality. One year, a few inspections ago, we were told that our patient information booklet was the best the inspectorate had come across. The chairperson of the inspecting team told us that this should be a model for other units in the country. We were even asked if we had any objection if parts of it might be used by the HFEA just for this purpose. One year later, at our next inspection, we were advised that the same booklet was misleading in some respects and that sections might not be fully intelligible. We were told that we should reprint it incorporating a number of amendments. This I was reluctant to do, on the grounds that reprinting a fairly thick booklet of that type would be prohibitively expensive. I was then asked to change the booklet at the earliest opportunity as soon as booklets from the current printing had run out. One year later, I confess we were still handing out the same booklet, and a third inspection team made flattering comments about the high standard of our patient information literature. While this is not particularly important, it clearly illustrates a serious lack of uniformity and objectivity on the part of HFEA inspection teams.

It would have been preferable for the HFEA to have established a more or less full-time fully trained inspection team. This is the system adopted by other official regulatory bodies. For example, the Home Office employs full-time professional inspectors to regulate research involving the use of animals. This ensures reasonably uniform decisions about licensing across the country and avoids the criticism of partiality or favouritism. No outsider can be certain why the HFEA did not take the decision to have a full-time inspectorate – possibly it was seen as an option which would be too costly. If this is the reason, it seems a poor one. Given the high standards that the HFEA continuously urge, and given that inspection of units is the most important aspect of their licensing work, it would seem essential that this work is above criticism. In any case the cost would not be so great – according to reasonable calculations it would now require a price increase of conservatively around £3 – £5 per patient licence fee.

Evaluating and regulation of some ethical issues

Sex selection

One of the difficult questions with which the HFEA had to wrestle early on, was that of sex selection. In 1993, two years after starting work, the Authority commenced public consultation on the ethical aspects of this issue. The way with which it was dealt showed both a strength and a limitation of the HFEA. Sex selection by removing cells from an embryo (preimplantation diagnosis) had already been successfully performed at The Hammersmith Hospital for those families which carry sex-linked disorders. The Authority stated that it had no problem in approving sex selection for such serious causes, but was concerned about sex selection for social reasons. After receiving over 200 responses to their most comprehensive consultation document, the HFEA carefully examined the issue. It published its findings later that year, pointing out that no new arguments beyond those in the document had surfaced. After these deliberations, it reported to the Government that it considered that sex selection purely for 'family balancing' or other social reasons was not justified.

But ironically, whilst these deliberations were in process, a commercial trade in sex selection was being conducted at a house in the UK. In spite of the HFEA's concerns, this clinic continued to practice – and as far as I am aware is still doing so some four years later. The practitioners in this clinic were using a method of 'sperm separation' which had been published some years earlier by a Dr Ericcson in the United States. This method involves passing the seminal fluid through a solution that acts as a kind of filter. Because sperm carrying the X chromosome ('female' sperm) are just marginally heavier than sperm carrying the Y chromosome ('male' sperm), it was stated that they would pass through such fluid at a slower rate. Claims have been made repeatedly that this form of sperm separation was fairly reliable, insemination with such enriched sperm suspensions giving a women a 70–80 per cent chance of having a baby of the desired sex. There is, however, very little evidence at all that the method works. After several years of what presumably must be quite a lucrative practice (several hundred pounds for each cycle of insemination) I am unaware of any properly evaluated results published by this clinic in a peer review journal. All this is ironic because insemination – provided it is not done using donor semen – is outside the law empowering the HFEA. By a curious loophole clinics like this do not appear to be regulated by any effective law. As I understand it, the person who has been running the clinic is not a medical doctor, but holds a PhD qualification so is legitimately able to call himself 'doctor'. It is widely believed that there is another retired doctor also involved, but as he is retired, he presumably is no longer registered with the General Medical Council (GMC). Consequently it would appear that the GMC, normally the doctors' regulatory body, would have little influence over practice at this clinic.

This paradox highlights one of the fundamental problems associated with the establishment of the HFEA. It was set up to regulate IVF and donor insemination, and areas of treatment where handling an early embryo is involved. It has no powers to regulate or oversee all other fertility and infertility treatments, for example tubal surgery, stimulation of ovulation, GIFT treatments (because they involve the introduction of unfertilised eggs to the tube – not embryos), abortion, contraception and management of miscarriage. In fact, the HFEA has no control over the great bulk of reproductive medicine.

It is perhaps pertinent to ask why *in vitro* fertilisation was singled out for such regulation. It certainly cannot be to improve clinical standards. Standards of tubal surgery are much more variable – there are some British units with less than five per cent of their patients getting pregnant after it, whilst others are achieving more than ten times that success due to better surgical technique and better patient selection. Nor can it be because IVF is more dangerous. Stimulation of ovulation without IVF is almost certainly the most dangerous of any reproductive treatment. It has a higher chance of high order multiple pregnancy (for example in the Mandy Allwood case, see page 170). Hyperstimulation has been more dangerous in those units with no IVF experience.

Payments to donors

Much of the time the HFEA has made important and really significant contributions to the debate about ethical issues. One recent example has been their response over the vexed question of payments to those donating eggs, sperm and embryos. There has always been public and parliamentary concern about paying donors for gametes or embryos. Indeed, this was something raised in the 1990 Act of Parliament. Quite early on in 1993, the HFEA implied that they might consider phasing out payments to all donors. It was already clear that sperm donors were largely motivated by the idea of a monetary payment but this appeared far less relevant for women who considered donating eggs. Women regard this largely as an altruistic act giving the pleasure and fulfilment of a child to another individual.

It was clear from their discussions that the HFEA wanted a just solution to this difficult problem. They did not want the supply of donated sperm and eggs to dry up. But they were also particularly concerned that potential donors should not be exploited. There was always the thought that people might be coerced into giving their eggs or sperm, only later to regret this act. In 1995 the HFEA held a conference in Oxford where they raised these issues. At that meeting serious consideration was given also to the need to provide better information to the general public. It was thought that if more publicity were given to the need for egg donors, that more women might come forward.

Since that time the HFEA has been increasingly concerned that payment to sperm and egg donors could jeopardise important ethical principles. They have been particularly worried that payment might be an unreasonable inducement and jeopardise the well-being of the donor. They also considered that payment for what was 'human life' in some way cheapened its value. It is true that donors of other tissues such as kidneys and blood, do not receive payment in the United Kingdom. Of course, the two are not synonymous because the donation of egg or sperm is in effect helping to create human life rather than to prevent death.

After a great deal of deliberation, the HFEA has concluded that donation should be a gift, freely and voluntarily given with informed consent. With that view in mind, it has come to the only logical conclusion possible – that payment to donors should be phased out. From this year, the only payments that can be made to donors are necessary and consequential expenses which have been incurred as an act of donation.

Throughout these deliberations, there was certainly a high moral tone about the HFEA's stand. Many doctors and scientists actually involved with donation have taken a much more pragmatic view, and some have been very critical of the HFEA. Many say that payment may recruit a financially motivated donor, but it does not alter the quality of the gamete produced. Some people have suggested that presentation of donation as a commercial transaction may actually attract the most suitable donors, with the right attitude for the job. They say that a detached and casual attitude by the donor, who is only interested in the money, means that there would be no fear of intrusion by the donor into the recipient family. Some Americans point out that all donation programmes would be impossible in the United States if it were not for relatively generous payment to donors. This may, regrettably, say much about attitudes in that great country. Dr Mark Sauer, from New York writes 'I am constantly asked, "Why pay donors?" I reply to those who ask, "Why not? . . . A lucrative industry has been built around sperm banking and has existed for decades, largely unquestioned." '

I am quite convinced that the HFEA's stance over this issue is correct. I think that it is necessary to be principled about issues which concern the creation of a child. It may be extremely inconvenient that more donors are not available. But inconvenience must not be the basis for these important decisions. There are many people who are increasingly concerned about the whole relationship between the unborn child and his anonymous donating parent. There is even a very good argument which suggests that all acts of donation should be registerable and identifiable. I think there may come a time when donors of gametes may have to accept responsibility for their genetic offspring. This is a very knotty question indeed but surely the HFEA is right not to cheapen the value of human life by allowing payment for it.

Fetal ovaries and donor eggs

But the HFEA miscued more significantly in the arena of egg donation four years ago. Then enormous press coverage was given to the idea that eggs suitable for donation might be retrieved from fetal ovaries. This was simply a theoretical idea put forward by the eminent reproductive scientist Professor Roger Gosden. He was not yet researching this possibility in humans, and had properly put the idea before an ethics committee to see what their reaction might be. As eggs are formed in the ovary well before birth and are held there in a state of arrest pending adulthood, Roger Gosden had argued that this might be worth considering as a good source of eggs for the treatment of women suffering from premature menopause. The fetal ovary is smaller than the adult ovary, and yet contains ten times more eggs than does the ovary of a mature woman. Here then was a huge concentration of eggs potentially ready for harvest providing methods could be developed for maturing those eggs outside the body. Perhaps predictably there was a wave of press and public reaction. Religious organisations – particularly those with strong views about abortion – were furious that doctors could apparently consider taking eggs from dead babies or, worse still, aborted fetuses.

The HFEA could have played an invaluable role by pointing out that this was only a research idea that was completely unfeasible. They could have said that even with the most intensive research it was likely to remain completely impossible for many years. Instead, without providing this context for debate, it started a public consultation process to see what various organisations and groups with an interest in the subject might feel. The effect was to encourage a wave of ill-informed press reports and public 'outrage'. The story gained momentum and it culminated in the introduction of a Parliamentary Bill calling for a ban on research involving human fetal ovaries. The then Secretary of State for Health, Mrs Virginia Bottomley supported the Bill, and fetal ovarian research was banned by the Knight amendment; a last minute addition to a Home Office Bill. It would have been far better if the Health Secretary had waited to hear the deliberation of her own appointed regulatory authority, the HFEA. To introduce hastily drafted legislation (which was completely unnecessary as nobody was even seriously considering such research) was to ensure inadequate discussion and reflection – and to limit potentially useful research.

The episode badly compromised the HFEA's standing. It would probably be much more effective in its declared aim of balancing public concern with scientific progress if it showed more understanding itself of the conditions that such scientific progress required. Without the intellectual freedom to speculate and hypothesise, scientists are powerless to pioneer treatments of genuine public benefit.

Discussions about cloning

Another area where HFEA involvement was probably unnecessary was over the issue of cloning. Cloning had been considered at length by a Select Committee of the House of Commons and subsequently by the Human Genetics Advisory Commission (HGAC). One cannot help wondering why the HFEA has chosen to give so much publicity to their own deliberations, which seem somewhat superfluous. More important to some people involved in IVF is the question about who paid for their report. Given that the HFEA seems very short of income one wonders why these deliberations were needed. The 1990 Act of Parliament makes it quite clear that nuclear transfer – the procedure needed to produce a clone – is illegal in humans. The report certainly brought the HFEA into ridicule in some quarters – in a wonderfully funny piece in *The Times* (9 December 1998) Simon Jenkins sums up his view:

'The writers of the HGAC/HFEA report may lack the style of Mary Shelley, but they know what stands the public's hair on end. They are near fanatical in their bans. Top of their list is anything to do with human reproduction . . .' and 'Regulators who pander to public terror of science will find the public duly terrified. Such a public will, in turn, terrorise the regulators . . . Britain is now the world capital of the ban. Whatever a minister, committee, newspaper or lobbyist finds distasteful is grist to the banning mill. If in doubt, ban it . . .'

I hasten to say that what they have said about it all is perfectly sensible (though I am reluctant to admit to a sneaking thought – would an infant really suffer simply because he or she carries only one parent's genetic identity?). Perhaps the most useful thing that comes out of their report is the recommendation that these technologies might be used for treatment for certain genetic diseases caused by the mitochondria, and for developing therapy for diseased or damaged tissues or organs.

Destruction of cryopreserved embryos

One episode which caused great controversy was when the HFEA, in 1996, authorised the destruction of embryos that had been cryopreserved for more than five years. The 1990 Act of Parliament had stipulated that embryos could not be held in frozen storage for five years. The Act came into force in 1991. It was a clear decision in what was an arbitrary period, but Parliament was simply reflecting widespread public concern regarding embryos that might be held in limbo indefinitely. The Act required that there should be informed written consent from each person who gives rise to the genetic material to be stored. But as the Chairman of the HFEA, Ruth Deech, correctly pointed out, whilst consent implies control, it does not involve ownership. Gametes and embryos cannot be 'owned'. Parliament did allow that there could be an extension to the statutory period of storage, providing the couples concerned gave further written signed consent.

There can be no doubt that everybody concerned with the cryopreservation of embryos knew that there was a five year deadline. Patients too, when consenting in writing, signed a form pointing out that their embryos were only preserved for five years. There was a clear indication to couples having their embryos frozen that they should keep clinics informed of a change of address should they require continued storage of embryos. Because the five year limit was running out, the HFEA was asked by the Department of Health in 1995 to produce a report on the issues surrounding the statutory period. This report was made public in Decembe 1995 and laid before Parliament two months later. The HFEA had secured approval for an extension of the time of freezing, providing the parents concerned had given signed consent in writing.

Now of course, there was a flurry of activity from the clinics who suddenly and belatedly tried to trace parents of embryos. But a number of genetic parents were completely untraceable, having moved address. Others did not reply to repeated postal enquiries.

On 1 August 1996, amidst a huge wave of press publicity, the destruction of time-expired embryos began. One has to say that the profession did not appear in a very good light. Earlier, some of my colleagues had been heard protesting volubly on television that they would rather go to prison than destroy these embryos. Others attacked the HFEA for their role in this matter. In the event, of course, no scientist was arrested because most of these statements were probably made more with the feeling of righteousness and self-publicity, than for any other reason.

Subsequently, in 1997, Professor Robert Edwards, the notable pioneer and 'father' of IVF, wrote summarising his feelings in the journal *Human Reproduction*:

> 'Embryologists in each IVF clinic consequently had to make up their minds . . . Many of them, although by no means all, did not wish to destroy the embryos and some refused to destroy them on ethical grounds . . . The HFEA countered by suggesting that another embryologist without such ethical scruples could undertake the task of destruction . . . Although this solution did nothing to remove the ethical objections to the wastage of such carefully preserved embryos, the HFEA remained adamant that the full force of law would be directed against any clinic failing to destroy its cohort of embryos . . . Last minute appeals for the HFEA . . . fell upon deaf ears. The liberal and imaginative attitude which had extended the five year period was for some reason lost with regard to the problems of parental consent for the use of spare embryos. For a period of time the HFEA became a different organisation to that we have known. Threats to take severe legal action against embryologists who wished to avoid the senseless destruction of embryos became a stock in trade, on television and elsewhere . . .'

I have to say that I am not particularly impressed by the emotive language used by Professor Edwards. I think it largely special pleading. What is interesting, is that there were virtually no cases of people who had left embryos in storage and who could not be traced at the time subsequently complaining about the decision. In any case, this was a piece of legislation which was widely known to the clinics concerned. They had been aware for five years that they would have to make provision for the removal of these embryos from storage. To suggest to the press as some doctors did at the time, that large numbers, possibly many thousands, of little human beings were being destroyed was probably more immoral than following the letter of the law. It was certainly more damaging to the reputation of our discipline.

I think the law was too rigid. I also think that Mrs Deech and the HFEA did its very best to make sure that as much common sense prevailed as possible. But we, as a profession did not do well. We were casual about frozen storage, and neglectful that the law would take its course. Above all, some of my colleagues demonstrated too few moral scruples and too much moral indignation.

Posthumous insemination, consent and Diane Blood

The Diane Blood case was different. It seemed to be an example of the HFEA's occasional tendency to place a narrow legalistic interpretation of its responsibilities before the interests of patients. In 1994, Mr and Mrs Blood decided to start a family. Not long afterwards Mr Blood contracted meningitis and became acutely ill. He was admitted to the intensive care of a Yorkshire hospital but rapidly deteriorated. At this time Mrs Blood had missed her period by just over a week and thought that she could be pregnant. She was concerned that her husband's illness would make him sterile and considered getting him to produce semen samples as a kind of insurance policy. Events moved very rapidly and with great confusion. Within hours of Stephen Blood's hospital admission he was in coma. After discussion with the doctors, semen was taken by electroejaculation so that it could be stored if necessary. The first sample was poor, so a repeat sample was taken some hours later. By this time Stephen was deeply unconscious and a few hours later he died. A few days later Diane had her period.

Unfortunately, Stephen died without giving written consent for sperm storage. At the time, the HFEA was contacted by telephone call to London and the senior person available agreed it would be cruel and unnecessarily beaurocratic to prevent the storage or destroy the sperm now that it was taken.

Months later, Diane Blood requested insemination with her dead husband's sperm. The unit contacted the HFEA who decided that it would not be legal for Mrs Blood to be inseminated with her husband's sperm because he had not consented in writing as was required by the 1990 Act of Parliament. The HFEA also refused to allow the export of the frozen sperm abroad so that Mrs Blood could receive treatment where UK law did not apply. To no avail, Mrs Blood claimed that she and her husband had a most serious commitment to having a family, and that they had discussed whether or not they would use assisted conception if necessary. She claimed (and later produced evidence) that they had even discussed what they would wish to happen should he die before she had had a conception. It was apparent from Mrs Blood's statements that she was a deeply religious Christian (as had been her husband) and that she regarded that in carrying out what she was convinced were Stephen Blood's wishes, she was completing the sacrament of her seven year marriage. In desperation, Mrs Blood's lawyers took her case to the High Court.

By this time Mrs Blood's case was something of a *cause célèbre*. Public opinion, whipped up by massive press coverage, was overwhelmingly in favour of allowing Mrs Blood her request, and what she effectively claimed were amongst her husband's last wishes. When the High Court found against Mrs Blood, she lodged an appeal. Finally, the Court of Appeal ruled that the HFEA was right to uphold the principle of written consent, but should have considered whether the 'public interest' was served when it decided to refuse the export of Mr Blood's sperm. The Court asked the HFEA to review its decision, and the Authority subsequently withdrew its objection to Mrs Blood's request for export. It required the intervention of an appeal court to suggest a degree of latitude and common sense that previously the HFEA had been unable to find.

Subsequently, Mrs Blood found a clinic in Belgium which treated her and her story after many months of real pain and unnecessary distress ended. In December 1998, Diane Blood gave birth to a little boy. In one sense she was a very lucky woman. Although she was a widow, she must have gained immense strength and courage for the really solid support given to her both by her family, and the family of her late husband.

Patient information

One of the responsibilities of the HFEA is to provide information about its regulatory procedures to Parliament, and general information about its service to prospective patients. It does this, in part, by providing an annual report, which is sent to the Secretary of State for Health, and which is subsequently published.

Its report is an excellent document and at the time of writing the Seventh Annual Report has been published. This year it reports that a total of 114 licensed clinics are now in operation of which 73 provide IVF, and the rest just donor insemination. The report gives up-to-date information about the HFEA's Code of Practice which it sends to all licensed centres, and which it updates regularly. As it points out, the HFEA has now published four editions of the Code of Practice, and is preparing a fifth edition.

A major concern in the Code of Practice are the considerations of the welfare of any child that might be born after IVF. This is a difficult and contentious area which the HFEA has dealt with in an exemplary fashion. It has tried exceptionally hard not to be unusually restrictive, and to show sound common sense and good judgement with regard to these issues.

The area of genetic testing also comes into the most recent Code of Practice and in particular, the HFEA is concerned about the screening of sperm donors for cystic fibrosis. As we have seen, cystic fibrosis is a common recessive disorder carried by between one in fifteen and one in twenty of the population. It will be all too easy to inseminate sperm from a carrier into a woman who is also a carrier, and run the risk of her having a child with cystic fibrosis.

One really major anxiety, which the HFEA underlines heavily in its report, is the issue of the large number of multiple births which occur in the UK as a result of IVF. In 1998, no fewer than 227 triplet or quadruplet pregnancies were engendered following IVF. This is a huge burden to the women bearing these multiple pregnancies, and costly for the NHS. Moreover, there is a high risk of abnormalities in these pregnancies and in the babies born. The use of ovulatory drugs for routine treatments not involving IVF is not licensed, therefore we do not have figures for the number of multiple births caused by these drugs overall. The total figure is, however, likely to be at least double that reported by the HFEA. In its report, the HFEA points out that a critical consideration is the number of embryos transferred, and it emphasises in its Code of Practice that it wishes to see as much restriction as is possible without unduly comprising treatment. There should be a broad consensus of agreement for this approach. There can be no doubt that attempting to induce a pregnancy in an infertile woman at all costs is simply undesirable and potentially dangerous.

The HFEA report to Parliament also presents in an excellent form the data that it has collected. The level of data collection is admirable and shows the HFEA in the best possible light. Indeed, I do not believe that there is another country in the world which could produce such solid statistics.

The report also deals with research conducted in the United Kingdom and some comments about its policy particularly with regard to issues like preimplantation diagnosis, cryopreservation, ICSI and some of the concerns of the Department of Health. Finally, as required by Parliament, the HFEA produces a detailed financial balance sheet each year. Although many clinicians and some patients have grumbled about the cost of the licence, I have no doubt that the HFEA spends its money extremely frugally. Indeed, it ought to get better funding than it does. I think a very strong case could be made for at least part of the extra funding coming from government, and a little extra on the licence fee would, for example, enable there to be a full-time, professional inspectorate.

The 'league tables'

At the same time that it publishes its report, the HFEA also publishes its *Patients' Guide to DI and IVF Clinics*. This document has some very sensible advice to patients and includes a brief survey of the licensed treatments with some suggestions about what patients may ask their doctor. It has a large section on issues which patients may wish to consider including problems concerned with multiple births, the risk of ovarian hyperstimulation, some tests and investigations to be done before IVF and so on. Together with its *Patients' Guide*, it encloses a breakdown of the results achieved by each clinic in the UK. These results include the pregnancy rate and the live birth rate per treatment cycle, per egg collection, and per embryo transfer.

The results for all clinics are published simultaneously in one booklet. Inevitably, comparisons will be made by so many interested parties and the press has pounced upon them as if they are a league table. The HFEA, and its Chairman Ruth Deech, have consistently denied that these results should be seen as such.

In spite of these protestations, it was inevitable that this was how they would be interpreted. Moreover, the HFEA reinforced that impression themselves. Until 1998, they have consistently applied a statistical adjustment to the results to try to make them comparable with each other. This adjustment was designed by statisticians employed by the HFEA. The adjustment tried to take into account the varying populations treated in each clinic precisely so that there could be some justified comparison between them.

There were two problems with this approach. Firstly this was a clear sign, that in spite of their protestations, the HFEA *was* publishing a 'league table'. Secondly, and ironically, the statistical adjustment was deeply flawed. The approach that the statisticians used was criticised by various people with statistical expertise but the HFEA seemed deaf to the criticisms. The precise method their statisticians used was never fully explained, and seemed arcane to most people used to analysing medical results. There was consistent denial that, for example, the cause of infertility made any difference to the results. This was clearly erroneous. It is now obvious from the latest statistics, published this year, that patients with tubal disease undoubtedly do significantly less well than patients suffering from any other kind of infertility. Such a factor makes a big difference if for example, a clinic is treating large numbers of patients with tubal disease and relatively few patients with endometriosis or male infertility. What is also misleading is that the HFEA's own records for cause of infertility are very poor. The HFEA has done little or nothing to improve reporting is this area. It is a constant concern to many patients who would like to have the security of having their infertility properly assessed and the cause understood.

As it happens, the notion that one could compare the results from different clinics was finally blown apart in the Summer of 1998. At that time, Doctors Marshall and Spiegelhalter published a detailed analysis in the *British Medical Journal* of the HFEA's data. They demonstrated clearly that any comparison between clinics was almost entirely flawed. It turns out, from their analysis, that there is virtually no statistical evidence of difference between any of the clinics in the country. The exception are just two clinics which are producing the worst UK results. It does seem that they are producing success rates which are statistically less good than the rest.

It is good that the *British Medical Journal* article was published when it was, but it came rather late. For some time, a number of senior clinicians have been trying to explain to the HFEA that there were problems with the way they had published these results:

First of all, as we have seen, a number of a factors make a significant difference to the chances of success. These include the age of patients treated in a particular clinic, the responsiveness of the ovaries found in a particular patient population (this undoubtedly varies very considerably from clinic to clinic), and the number of treatment cycles the patients have previously had before entering the programme in a particular clinic. At The Hammersmith Hospital, over the last three years for example, something like four-fifths of the new patients I have seen personally in my own clinic have already failed an average of two to three IVF attempts in other clinics. This inevitably depresses the success rate we can achieve.

There is also the vexed question of the number of embryos transferred. Though this makes much less difference to live birth rates, there is no doubt that some clinics take considerable risks in transferring more than two embryos in relatively young patients. One of the problems about publishing a comparative table of results is that it encourages clinics to take these risks because clearly they want to be seen to be doing better than their rivals. IVF is, unfortunately, a commercial business. Even in the health service, there is the need to satisfy NHS purchasers and they pay probably too much attention to these results.

One of the biggest problems about league tables is that their publication encourages some clinics unreasonably to exclude women whose prognosis is unfavourable. Exclusion of the women least likely to benefit will improve the results gained by a clinic but it is unfair. It deprives many deserving women whose only chance of having a baby is IVF. We are seeing an increasing number of women in this situation, who are not even being given the privilege of trying. Failure of IVF can also be a kind of success – somebody who has tried everything and failed may find it much easier to come to terms with their infertility.

The pressure to be high in the league table also inhibits research. As we have seen throughout this book, one of the greatest problems facing improvements in IVF is the lack of good, properly controlled trials to test different treatments. Conducting a controlled trial is inevitably going to affect a clinic's results adversely. When two treatments are being compared, one group of patients is likely to do less well than another group. But this implies depressing the results which are reported to the HFEA. Exactly the same applies to treatments like genetic screening by preimplantation diagnosis. These treatments can never have quite as good a success rate; clinics that offer them are inevitably likely to depress their overall success.

A very serious problem with league tables is that their presence undoubtedly encourages a few clinics to be 'somewhat economical with the truth'. Some IVF clinics prematurely abandon cycles which look like being unsuccessful, and convert them to GIFT or to IUI. As neither of these latter treatments are regulated, and therefore not reported to the HFEA, these failures will not appear on the clinic's returns. There is also the inevitable thought that clinics may actually cheat when they make returns. There is no evidence that this has happened, but there is always the concern that it might in future.

Finally, one of the problems with the reported results is that they are published almost two years later. The results from individual clinics, only represent the results that they were getting 24 months, or even longer ago. As we have seen from annual reports from different clinics, a clinic can easily be top of the league one year, and not be far from the bottom in another year. This can make it very difficult for a perfectly honest and highly competent clinic to compete when there is an unavoidable commercial component to this improperly funded treatment.

As stated, the HFEA has repeatedly claimed that it is not producing league tables but these published results are certainly perceived as such. The HFEA has a statutory duty to maintain adequate public information, as laid down by Parliament. The current way of reporting results does to some extent misinform patients, and therefore damages their interest in various different ways. It is clear that a re-evaluation of how results are reported needs to be made. It is good that the HFEA has, during 1998, for the first time published UK success rates in an undirected form without any statistical comparison or statistical weighting. It is, I think, an unspoken admission that they need to consider an improvement. They have called this the *Interim Patients' Guide to DI and IVF Clinics*. To some people, it will seem curious that it has taken six years to get around to publishing an 'interim guide'.

Do we need a regulatory body?

I, like many colleagues, was highly enthusiastic about the formation of the HFEA. Now, after seven years of experience, I confess to having some nagging doubts about its role. As I have said, it does seem illogical to single out just one kind of medical treatment – not even the whole of reproductive medicine – for such careful, elaborate regulation. There have been occasions, too, when in spite of its role to educate and inform, the HFEA has appeared less than well-informed.

Regulators are bound, by their very nature, to have a kind of dominant gene for being stubborn. This is an unattractive trait and one that can prevent consensus. I hope that our regulators continue to demonstrate flexibility and wisdom. Over the next few decades, reproductive medicine is going to open out in ways that can be only remotely predicted at present. We have only just touched on the issues. It is difficult to think of what could happen for example with gene engineering if, on a global scale, there is not better regulation. Across the Atlantic, the USA is a free-for-all. It resists any regulation and that is the worst possible example to the world in general. The HFEA, by obtaining consensus and by demonstrating that regulation can work to everybody's advantage, could play a part as a major paradigm for the best way forward. Let us hope that it is up to this most difficult task.

9
Ethical dilemmas

Resources

Only a fraction of couples who might benefit from IVF actually do. In spite of the existence of the National Health Service, IVF is by and large a treatment for those who can afford to pay for it. Probably less than ten per cent of IVF in Britain is done through the NHS. Nor do private medical insurance companies, such as BUPA and PPP to their eternal shame, fund any part of IVF treatment. Indeed in Britain it is increasingly difficult to get any advanced fertility treatments on a free basis, even though we are repeatedly told by successive governments that theirs is the 'Government of family values'.

The great hurdle for infertile couples is the widespread attitude that infertility is not a real health problem. One local health authority recently considered ceasing to fund fertility treatment in response to a local survey which showed that most people saw such treatment as the lowest health priority. The situation is not dissimilar in some parts of the United States. A newsletter of the American support group Resolve noted that infertility treatment was ranked 602nd in importance in a list of 709 medical treatments compiled by the State of Oregon. This attitude is, fortunately, by no means typical of all American states. At least in America, most private insurers (unlike our British ones) recognise the need to fund these treatments.

The trouble is that unless you have suffered from infertility yourself it is extraordinarily difficult to understand the misery that this disease process can cause. Although we may not hear of people dying from infertility, it is none the less a condition which causes most of its victims extraordinary pain, a pain which is private and difficult to express (and therefore to resolve) because it is so personal.

We often hear, of course, that in an ideal world it would be a very good idea to fund IVF on the NHS. However, people go on to say, we do not live in an ideal world and there is only a finite amount of money available. The problem is, it is said, that while people are dying of kidney failure and we need to make increasing provision for our ageing population, it is not justified to spend more money on trivial medical conditions such as infertility. Now, I am not asking for a great expansion of public expenditure on health care, although it is true that we spend less per capita on health in Britain than most European countries. What I do argue is that we could spend what we are spending much more prudently.

Private funding from public funds

The NHS is still living with the legacy of the last government – the internal market – although it is welcome news that the present administration has pledged to abolish it. This method of health provision has led to considerable injustice in the case of infertile couples. The internal market requires local health authorities to provide health care for residents in the area of the country for which they are responsible. They are given a budget and committees within the health authorities (the purchasers) decide whether to buy particular services, and from which clinics or hospitals. The result is that whether an infertile couple receives NHS treatment or not is a completely arbitrary matter, a question of where they happen to live. According to a recent report, Scottish health authorities paid for 27 IVF treatments for every 100,000 people compared with less than four treatments per 100,000 in the South and West of England. In Northern Ireland, no provision is made for infertility treatment at all.

Not only does the internal market result in such a patently unfair division of the taxpayer's investment in health care, but also it has resulted in considerable wastage of money. The 'providers' are the general hospitals who tender to provide a particular service under contract, be it IVF or general surgery, for a given number of patients from that health authority. Organisations other than the general hospitals can also tender for contracts.

In the case of IVF, many of the larger private clinics are competing for contracts within the health service. Sometimes the private clinics have offered their services under contract at quite a high price, certainly higher than many NHS or university hospital providers. Even so purchasers have taken up contracts with them when they could have been re-investing their money in the NHS. These decisions to opt for a particular private clinic were sometimes made for rather curious reasons. There are instances of contracts being signed because of a favourable geographical location close to the purchasing authority when it might have been better for couples to travel. Sometimes purchasing authorities (who generally have had a poor understanding of the intricacies of IVF and the interpretation of the results that a given clinic may be advertising) are bemused by the apparently favourable information that a private clinic is putting out. Some private clinics spend considerable sums of money on promotional material which looks extremely enticing except perhaps to the most discerning reader. Purchasers buying IVF from a private clinic may well be paying more than they might from a good district hospital, and the funds that the private clinic receives are basically turned back into profits for the clinics' shareholders. The net result is a drop in investment in the public sector, which has several undesirable consequences.

Most of the good scientific progress has always traditionally been made in the public sector in this country, and still is. In the IVF field a survey of published research shows that the public (especially the university) sector has been much more scientifically prolific, which suggests that most useful innovation in the field comes from these centres. Although there are far more private clinics than NHS ones, it is interesting that less than ten per cent of licences for basic research granted by the HFEA are registered in private clinics. The bulk of the important research papers and nearly all the peer review grants – the yardstick of research achievement – are in the public sector. When the health authorities purchase medical treatment from private clinics they are spending money which in the public sector would go much further towards supporting progress in the field.

Competition rather than centralisation

One of the principles underlying the internal market was that competition would drive prices down. But there has been little evidence of this happening in the health care 'market'. In the IVF field more and more small units have opened up in competition with each other. NHS general hospitals with minimal expertise, casting around for new areas to market, latched on to IVF, sometimes seen as a particularly rewarding area because it is apparently so profitable in the private sector. The competition that developed around The Hammersmith Hospital was an example. London already had over twenty IVF units – more than enough to cope with any demand. Hammersmith had one of the biggest in London, with a staff of 80, and the equivalent of four specialist consultants. It provides the whole range of infertility treatment – for example our success rate for tubal surgery is one of the best in the world, yet most of the time operating theatres are empty because we cannot get patients. With regard to IVF, the comprehensive large units are often likely to be more successful than small units, because there is a greater concentration of expertise, better staffing levels, more experience and better laboratories in large units.

A few years ago a new IVF unit opened in an NHS hospital, within a few miles of The Hammersmith Hospital. This hospital had no specialist infertility clinic and, as far as I am aware, had published little in this scientific area in recent years. It had no specialist fertility consultants and certainly could not then provide truly comprehensive infertility care. When asked how they intended to compete with The Hammersmith Hospital and its world-class facilities, the reply was: 'We intend to undercut their prices.'

This would actually be quite difficult to do. The Hammersmith Hospital amasses considerable charitable funding and private income is channelled back into the NHS system. It is actually one of the cheaper units in the country – let alone London, which tends to be a more expensive city than average. So the result is another IVF unit in London which is probably unnecessary. Eventually this unit is likely to become unprofitable and close (or amalgamate with its neighbours) after considerable NHS resources have been spent commissioning it and maintaining its staff.

I must emphasise that I am not against private IVF. Most private units in Britain are excellent and would bear comparison with any in the world. But most private IVF clinics are free-standing; that is to say, they are IVF units pure and simple, not often set up to conduct comprehensive fertility care. In such places, IVF is bound to be offered routinely because it is much simpler for the clinic to conduct such treatments. Patients attending some of them are increasingly at risk of getting the most convenient rather than the most appropriate treatment. Leaving aside potentially unnecessary treatment and the issue of the amount of likely distress that may be caused, all this is wasteful of resources.

Wastage of NHS resources

An example of wastage of resources is the unnecessarily high drugs bill that the decentralisation of NHS provision has caused. A cycle of IVF can cost anything from £1,400–£2,400, but this figure does not include the cost of drugs needed to make the ovaries produce several eggs at once, nor treatments like ICSI to enhance fertilisation. The drugs used to stimulate the ovaries are made up in glass ampoules. Each ampoule costs between £10–£30 and usually an average of 30 are needed. Many patients need 60 or more ampoules with a retail cost of perhaps £2000. Consequently most clinics ask patients to get their drugs supplied on prescription from their GP. In the case of NHS patients, this saves hospital pharmacies from prescribing from their hard-pressed drug budget. In the case of private clinics, this reduces the overall cost to the patient, who may get her drugs from a GP sympathetic to her plight; however, this is entirely haphazard. Moreover, it adds greatly to the drug bill that the taxpayer eventually has to pay. This is because hospitals get drugs direct from the manufacturer at the basic price, often with a discount. By contrast, GP prescriptions are sold by retail pharmacists in the high street and there is usually a considerable mark-up. An ampoule costing £10 in the hospital pharmacy may cost twice or even more when dispensed over the counter of the local chemist's shop. Consequently 30 ampoules which might cost £300 if given by a hospital could cost the NHS at least £600. It is likely that at least an extra £5 million is spent in Britain in this way annually – enough to give another 5,000 patients one chance at IVF on an NHS basis in NHS hospitals where most offer this treatment on a contract basis.

Avoidance of fragmentation of care

Unfortunately, even with the abolition of the internal market I fear that there could still be fragmentation of health care. The consequences are still that there will be less effective treatment, or treatments of all sorts with less expertise. At present it is uncertain whether infertility will be under the responsibility of the Primary Care Groups – essentially general practitioner driven, or whether they will be under the specialist medicine provided by local authorities in the various regions. In the field of infertility I believe we could provide a far better organised and efficient service, to more patients, without any extra spending at all. One of the greatest gains of the present government's intention to abolish the internal market will be the centralisation of resources for such treatments as IVF. Regional services in major centres would be a much better investment for the taxpayer. Considerable expertise could be concentrated there, and the bigger throughput would ensure much more efficient and cheaper medical care. Given proper thought, patients could still experience individualised IVF where there was a high degree of personal care. The rationalisation of space, materials and staffing would ensure the best value for money. It would also ensure the best chance of a pregnancy. Certainly it is true that a couple may need to travel a little further for their treatment, but at the end of the journey they would have the confidence of being offered the best IVF available.

The following is an example of the misery that our present haphazard system of provision can cause: nearly two years ago, on the fiftieth anniversary of the foundation of the National Health Service, Lucy and John, a happily married couple, came to ask my advice. Eight years previously when she was just 25 years old, Lucy had gone to her GP because she had been trying for a baby for almost two years. Her GP did not examine her but referred her to a private gynaecologist in Harley Street. The gynaecologist, who was not an infertility specialist, found a large lump in her uterus, the size of a twenty-week pregnancy. He diagnosed this correctly as a benign tumour – a fibroid. He advised immediate surgery, reassuring Lucy that the operation was routine. Not only did he not do any further investigations, beyond testing for Lucy's blood group, but more importantly, he took no steps to shrink the tumour first by giving his patient a short course of hormones. This is routinely done by experienced surgeons because it makes surgery easier and less likely to be complicated. The operation was conducted at a small private clinic. There was considerable blood loss and the procedure was a prolonged struggle. Lucy, being young and fit rapidly started to recover. However, on the fourth day after the operation, she suddenly felt very unwell and collapsed. A second, much bigger blood transfusion was given, and she was rushed back to theatre. Her surgeon re-opened her abdomen and repaired the bleeding wound in her uterus, which had broken apart, after being inadequately stitched four days earlier.

Lucy went home seven days later, weak but reasonably well and reassured that it should be a simple matter for her to conceive now everything had been corrected. Three years later Lucy was still not pregnant. The gynaecologist advised there was nothing further he could do and suggested IVF. Her GP referred her to a private clinic run by a contemporary at the same medical school. It was geographically distant, but there was no waiting list. Six weeks later, after paying in advance for private IVF, a course of drugs was given to stimulate her ovaries – these could be prescribed on the NHS and cost almost £1,000. Unfortunately, Lucy over-responded to them. Hyperstimulation is a painful and agonising process but Lucy and John were thrilled that eleven eggs had been collected under a general anaesthetic. Unfortunately, none fertilised – John had a sperm problem which had not been diagnosed beforehand.

Not surprisingly, John and Lucy, though generally very optimistic people, felt disillusioned. Both teachers, the money they had spent so far was significant. Nonetheless, having children of their own was by far their first priority, and they felt that a more expensive clinic would give them better care. At the new clinic, the consultant was breezy. He suggested that it might be worthwhile to do laser surgery to clear any adhesions after her original operation. The surgery cost around £2,500 and recovery was swift. After it, the consultant was somewhat less sanguine – one tube, he said, was hopelessly damaged following removal of the fibroid. He suggested further IVF treatment at his clinic. Another two IVF cycles with more careful monitoring this time, at a cost of £3,500 each, produced embryos. Remembering John's problem, individual sperm were injected into each egg. Three embryos were transferred to the uterus at each treatment. Sadly, Lucy did not conceive and here she was sitting in my clinic, still smiling, still optimistic.

When John and Lucy left my clinic after telling me all this, I was genuinely close to tears – due to anger and frustration. Frustration because all this treatment would have been available at an excellent NHS hospital four miles from her house. And anger because her menstrual symptoms strongly suggested that her uterine cavity was almost certainly severely damaged by the original operation. No doctor had thought to do a simple inexpensive X-ray before IVF treatment. Their embryos had been produced and transferred with little or no chance of a pregnancy.

Each month I see dozens of patients with similar stories of incomplete diagnosis and inappropriate treatment. Some are not quite as bad, but others are worse. The one consistent pattern is that, because of lack of NHS provision – due to lack of funding – more and more ordinary men and women, people who never would normally consider private health care, are forced into the private sector. Much of the time private care is excellent, but it is always expensive. Consequently many private clinics do fewer investigations. Often they offer the treatment at which they are best, rather than the most appropriate one.

Three years ago the distressing case of Mandy Allwood was in the headlines. She had conceived octuplets after taking fertility drugs. She rejected medical advice that she should have some of the fetuses aborted in order to increase the survival chances of the remainder. In the event she lost all eight babies, and a furious debate raged in the newspapers over the medical and ethical issues involved. Some thought that a patient should not be allowed to ignore medical advice when such serious consequences would almost certainly ensue; others that the selective abortion the doctors advised was an infringement of the rights of the unborn child. In the aftermath some doctors refused to prescribe fertility drugs for their patients, and other infertile couples had to pay a price for the exceptional circumstances of the Mandy Allwood case. This tendency to stigmatise fertility treatments was all the more regrettable because the case was really yet another example of the inadequacy of NHS provision. If IVF research were properly supported, the treatment would be less than half the cost, and its wider availability would reduce the need for commercial clinics to prescribe infertility drugs – often causing multiple births and complications. Indeed, the option of IVF would have saved the NHS the thousands of pounds spent dealing with the complications that arose from Mandy Allwood's multiple pregnancy, as well as considerable grief and heartbreak. When it was found that she had produced so many eggs, they could have been fertilised *in vitro* with her partner's sperm. Two embryos could then have been transferred back to the uterus, and the remainder saved for future transfer.

Rationing

Centralisation of health care provision would make it possible to introduce an equitable and consistent system of rationing and a proper assessment of whether a patient's medical condition warrants IVF. There should certainly be nationally accepted guidelines for when NHS IVF treatment should be considered. At present the criteria of eligibility is as arbitrary as whether a particular Health Authority will offer IVF in the first place. There are differing limits about the age of patients accepted, the number of treatment cycles funded and the existence of children already produced by that partnership. One of the problems is that there is a whole range of social issues which complicate the availability and suitability of IVF treatment. When IVF first started there were very serious discussions about whether IVF should be made available to couples who are living together but not formally married. Most people would now think this entirely acceptable, but by no means everybody. If a couple is living together, should there be a minimum time-limit on how long they should cohabit in order to ensure that they are genuinely in a stable relationship? At first this may seem rational and fair, but it is worth considering that the fertile members of the population do not have to go through any such assessment when they are considering having a baby.

Health authorities are very reluctant to offer IVF treatment to women over 40 because they see this as a treatment much more likely to be wasted. Sometimes the decision is even more questionable. In 1995, the Health Authority in Sheffield decided that it would not offer NHS funding for an IVF treatment for a woman, Mrs F., aged 37. Their decision appeared to be taken mostly on the grounds that, given her age, treatment was less likely than average to succeed and therefore the money would not be well spent. Mrs F. appealed to the courts, but her application to get funding was refused and the decision of the Health Authority ratified.

It is worth taking a look at this decision. In our unit at that time given the then selection of cases, a woman of 37 would have had a 23 per cent chance of having a baby with one IVF cycle; a woman of 36 a 25.5 per cent chance. The difference of less than two per cent was, effectively, the difference between funding or not funding. Suppose, instead of being 37 years old, Mrs F. had been 35 years old and two stone overweight. Her chances of getting pregnant would have been about fourteen per cent – almost half the normal chance for a woman of 35 and substantially less than a woman of 37. Yet she would have been regarded as completely acceptable for NHS treatment in Sheffield, and probably in nearly every Health Authority in Britain that is prepared to offer this treatment.

One of the biggest issues is whether a couple should be offered IVF when they have already had a child in that relationship. Most purchasing authorities are extremely reluctant to consider arranging IVF via the NHS under such circumstances. Yet for many women the distress of infertility is as acute when they have had one child as it is when they had no children. Many families also feel very concerned about bringing up an only child if this can be avoided.

Welfare of the unborn child and autonomy of patients

The situation is particularly difficult for single women. The 1990 Act of Parliament and the HFEA's Code of Practice stipulate that the welfare of any child born as a result of IVF should be considered when clinicians embark on IVF treatments. Where there is no legal father it states: 'Centres are required to have regard to the child's need for a father and should pay particular attention to the prospective mother's ability to meet the child's needs throughout their childhood.' From time to time we are asked to provide treatment for single women – for example, with stored frozen sperm after a husband's death – or treatment for a lesbian couple. At first, it would seem that this is a perfect example of where a child is likely to be disadvantaged. No father figure exists and there is no male sex role model. It is widely believed that children brought up by a lesbian couple may exhibit some profound sexual disturbance. As it happens, there is no serious evidence that children born to single women or lesbian couples are in any way disadvantaged. Most of the studies which have been done on single-parent families are studies under various conditions of deprivation. There have been no definitive long-term studies of cases where single women could clearly afford to maintain a much-wanted child, or where a lesbian couple was happily providing the parenting required.

It is an impossible burden for clinics and the staff working in them to make judgements about the welfare of unborn children and therefore, by implication who is suitable to have children. Of course, there are the rare clear-cut cases. Families with a criminal history of persistent child abuse have almost certainly lost their right to find infertility treatment. But in most circumstances, there is a worrying fear that doctors are being asked to take authoritarian decisions which may be based mostly on their own prejudices. Of course, nobody wants to see a child being engendered in a desperately unhappy environment. But perhaps the bottom line is the question asked by Dr Raanan Gillon, the noted ethicist. He asks the question 'Is it better to have been born, than never to have been born at all?' I, for one, do not know the answer.

An important ethical principle in making decisions about offering IVF treatment is respect for the autonomy of people seeking it. I am often faced with particularly desperate couples for whom the only chance of a baby is IVF, but for whom the chance even with this treatment is very poor. I know that in their case IVF is unlikely to succeed because of the medical circumstances. I may also feel, perhaps knowing the couple who are seeking private treatment, that IVF could be too great a financial or psychological burden for them. Nevertheless, ultimately it would be wrong for me to refuse this couple treatment once they are in the position of knowing all the facts. They surely have the right to choose. If their autonomy is to be properly respected, the couple must be given all the information possible and then left free to decide for themselves.

I can think of only two exceptions to this principle. Firstly, a dictum about medical treatment should be that, wherever possible, it does no harm and potentially may do good. Doctors choosing which patients to treat by IVF must first consider the adverse consequences. It seems to me that I would be absolutely right to refuse treatment to a couple if I thought that the risks to their health very greatly outstripped the possible benefits. If I feel deeply uncomfortable about treating a couple, then my own autonomy is also deserving of respect. I believe I would also be justified in withholding treatment in the situation where I, as the doctor, have strong suspicions that any child born might be seriously at risk.

Treating older women

I have serious misgivings about treating women much after the natural menopause. These concerns were highlighted a couple of years ago by the case of Elizabeth Buttle, the 60-year-old woman who with the help of fertility treatment, gave birth to a son after lying about her age. It seems to me that there are very good reasons why treating women in their late 50s or early 60s is undesirable, and potentially very harmful. Irrespective of the patient's autonomy, first is concern for the woman herself. Pregnancy and childbirth, not to say early child nurture, are demanding for all parents, but obviously more burdensome for the woman. Statistics show that maternal deaths are much more likely in pregnant women in later childbearing years. A woman of 40 plus has a tenfold increased risk of death in pregnancy compared with a woman in her 20s. This is not such a great risk, admittedly, because death associated with pregnancy is nowadays a very rare event. Nevertheless, this risk will be higher still in a woman of 50 or 60 – indeed, because successful pregnancy is so rare in this age group, we can only merely guess at the relative risk involved. The risk, though, is not only that of death, but a more general and important one of serious ill-health.

High blood pressure, and hence toxaemia of pregnancy, are much more likely in women bearing children in later years. Diabetes, too, is much more likely because of the strain that pregnancy puts on the metabolic system. These diseases of pregnancy are dangerous for the mother – frequently necessitating prolonged hospital care and possibly damaging the health of the woman concerned – and they also affect the developing infant. Older mothers are prone to give birth to small, growth-retarded babies, especially if serious disease occurs in pregnancy. Consequently, there is a greater risk of loss of the baby before, during and after delivery.

Other physical risks to older mothers include heart disease, particularly heart attacks. After the menopause a woman's arteries start to harden and she develops the same risk of coronary thrombosis as a man. Treatment with oestrogens on a short-term basis – for example, to get a woman pregnant – will not reverse this, and the immense increase in the blood volume and extra work the heart has to do during pregnancy make heart attack a possibility. Another potential killer is venous thrombosis. Older women are much more prone to develop blood clots in the veins which can become dislodged by mere movement of the body and block off the blood supply to a lung. Sudden death by pulmonary embolus may follow. A clot can also enter the circulation of the brain and cause a stroke. These risks are also more likely in women having operative delivery such as a Caesarean section, an operation incidentally that older pregnant patients are three times more likely to need.

There are also serious risks of psychological or emotional damage. In order to understand this, we need to consider why a women in her late 50s or early 60s might feel such desperation for a child, at almost any cost. Why might she be prepared to lie to obtain treatment, for example? There is considerable evidence that many such women are actually going through a protracted bereavement process. They are mourning not only their lack of a child but also the ageing process which brings with it the cessation of the ability to procreate. Perhaps there are similarities with those cases of desperate women stealing babies from prams in supermarkets.

Such a pronounced grief reaction, possibly unrecognised by an infertility clinic, can result in a huge emotional backlash. When such a woman finally manages to find a doctor who is prepared to treat her, she is buoyed up with even more fraught emotions. She enters the hurdle race of IVF, with failure the probable outcome. Any underlying state of depression or grief surfaces once again, but in a much more intense form. Worse still, a grieving woman in this situation may become pregnant, but miscarry – an event which in any case is more likely in older women. The shock of a pregnancy loss, no matter how early on, in a woman who is already disturbed or depressed can be catastrophic. I will always remember one such case from the early days of my work with IVF. A 46-year-old woman who was desperate, literally pleaded for us to treat her. Her very desperation made us all uneasy but made it difficult to be rational about her – we simply did not have the heart to refuse. After she failed to get pregnant she tried to commit suicide on two occasions, before forced admission to a psychiatric institution where she spent the next two years.

It must also be considered whether treatment of older mothers is in the interest of the child. An older woman is likely to have less energy to devote both to pregnancy and subsequently to caring for the baby. The chore of getting up for night feeds, of being on call throughout the day, and the constant attention that a growing toddler needs as he or she explores their surroundings, place considerable demands on parents. A woman giving birth at 60 will be 70 years old before the child is even a teenager, by which time the child is not unlikely to be an orphan. The embarrassment of children of much younger elderly parents at being taken to school by their 'grandmother' is well documented. Such a child, possibly an only child in view of parental infertility, will be denied much of the usual physical stimulus that is the prerogative of normal childhood. Parents in their 70s are unlikely to be adequate goalkeepers in the back garden.

One frequently heard argument in favour of treating older women is that to not do so is in some way sexist. Men are fertile well into their 70s; Picasso was a father when over 80. There is surely, though, a difference between male and female parenting. This is not a sexist attitude, but in most societies, certainly even in our so-called advanced western society, the female partner generally plays a much more crucial role in rearing children.

One of the serious arguments against treating post-menopausal women in this way concerns the views of the egg donor. A woman who is post-menopausal can only conceive if she receives an egg from another woman. Compared to post-menopausal recipients, donors are much younger women. In England, regulation requires that they are under 35 years old, to reduce any risk of a genetic defect such as Down's syndrome in any resulting child. Donors go through considerable inconvenience and some risk to donate eggs, which are, of course, their own unique genetic material. What rights should they have in deciding who gets this precious gift? This is an important issue when the recruitment of egg donors is so very difficult.

When we at The Hammersmith Hospital have asked donors how they felt about their eggs going to much older woman, the reaction has usually been one of concern. They are less inclined to go through the demanding donation procedure if they are unhappy about the recipients of their generosity. As caring and sympathetic people, they feel compassion for those who, in later life, remain childless. But as rational human beings, they would rather see the chance of pregnancy go to someone fitter and healthier, with a greater chance of seeing the child safely into adulthood. Their act of donation is, psychologically at least, not without strings.

In this country it seems that altruistic donors see their eggs going to women with whom they can identify closely, and to potential families similar to their own ideals. Perhaps donors should have some say in how their eggs are 'distributed'. Pragmatism argues that doctors should be cautious about who receives donated eggs, otherwise supplies may dry up. This is already happening in the United States. Considerable press publicity was given to one particular IVF clinic in New York, and another in Los Angeles. Both clinics had made a considerable reputation treating postmenopausal women using donated eggs. Neither clinic was reticent about its treatment and featured prominently on television and in the newspapers. In the commercial atmosphere that surrounds aspects of American medical care, it is not necessarily to the financial disadvantage of a private clinic (and in the USA even university clinics are run on a private basis) to be prominent in the media. Great publicity was given to the policy of treating older women, but the supply of altruistic donors from the general public dried up almost totally. Eggs now used in most donor programmes in the USA are so-called 'spare' eggs from other IVF patients' treatment cycles.

All this leads me to raise what I feel is my most powerful objection to treating women who are well over 50. Most members of the public think it a misuse of technology, and some find it abhorrent. Whether or not they are right to feel as they do is, in a sense, irrelevant. When at the cutting edge of any new technology, its protagonists must take public opinion into account when considering what is ethical and therefore acceptable. IVF is a privileged and precious technology, poorly funded and, at the moment, largely the province of people who are somewhat better off financially than average. It is also a powerful technology, demonstrating what is possible in medicine. It has a great potential for human good, particularly as we unravel some of the mysteries of human genetics. To bring it into public disrepute would be to jeopardise that powerful but delicate technology. What limited funding is available may dry up, and important research about the very basis of human life might be curtailed. That would be too high a price to pay for the right to treat a few older women whose right to this risky therapy is, at best, arguable.

There is also an interesting medical principle here. It is the issue of when a treatment ceases to be for medical reasons, and is being used for social ones. Most people would have little concern over treating young women with premature menopause which has been brought on by cancer treatment. The use of donor eggs in these cases, as it is in young women whose ovaries just stop functioning in their 20s or 30s, seems quite justified. When we treat such women we are treating them for what is clearly defined as a pathological and therefore 'unnatural' condition. It seems to me though that women in their 50s or 60s are not having treatment for a diseased state, but rather for social reasons.

The HIV-positive patient

The treatment of infertile patients with HIV offers a contrasting example. However many difficult issues such treatment may raise, it seems to me to have a fundamental justification. The chief dilemma for a doctor should be one of weighing up the medical risks and the welfare of the people involved.

A few years ago I had to decide whether or not to treat a woman, whom I shall call Sheila. She was HIV-positive and therefore at risk of developing AIDS at a later date. At nineteen, Sheila had been a heroin user and was heavily under the influence of a boyfriend who almost certainly infected her with the HIV virus. Some years later she escaped her boyfriend's clutches and overcame her drug addiction. When we first met, she had been free of any drugs for eight years, and HIV-positive for ten. For the last five years she had been in a totally supportive relationship. Because they knew that she was HIV-positive, the couple had been practising safe sex since they had met. Her partner was free of the virus. Although they were not married, their relationship was clearly very stable. Both of them desperately wanted children and they came to consult me about their infertility, the result of Sheila having blocked tubes.

The three of us, Sheila, Alan and I, went over the arguments for and against IVF. Against treatment was the idea that Sheila was eventually likely to contract AIDS and die of the disease. Her child could be motherless within a year or two of birth. Then there was a finite possibility that the baby could be born with this infection, and could also die within a few years of birth. It was difficult to get an accurate estimate of the risk of the baby being born infected, but there might have been a eight to twelve per cent risk. To some extent this risk could be kept in check by not allowing the baby to be born vaginally and doing a Caesarean section instead. With this and by giving antiviral drugs during pregnancy, the risk of transferring the virus might be kept to around seven per cent. However, nobody I had carefully consulted beforehand could give a clear indication of the precise risk.

In favour of treatment was the knowledge that many people have children knowing there may be reasons why they may die in the near future. Many others quite responsibly have children knowing that, because they carry a gene for a fatal inherited disease, their baby may have a 50 per cent chance of dying within a year or so of birth. This is a gamble they take – as I believe they are entitled to take – in the hope of having normal offspring. There was also the knowledge that some people who are HIV-positive remain so for very extended periods of time, without necessarily developing full-blown AIDS. Sheila had been completely well for ten years with a normal blood count, and might remain well for very much longer. But above all, there was my increasing impression after four lengthy out-patient sessions that Sheila and Alan were highly responsible and caring people, who loved each other, who had thought it all through and wanted the chance of a baby. It was clear that had Sheila been normally fertile, she and her partner would not be sitting in front of me requesting my permission for IVF, for which they wanted to pay. I was sure that I should respect their autonomy.

I was not required to do so but I presented my interest in this case to the HFEA. Not only did the HFEA raise no objection, but they were positively helpful and open-minded. While the HFEA was worried about the complex problems involved, it felt that this was ultimately the kind of decision which had to be taken by the doctor together with the patients themselves. The Chairman of our Ethics Committee was in favour of treatment, as indeed were several senior colleagues with whom I raised the issue. But some members of my team initially expressed their extreme hostility to the idea, and it was only many months later, after much further discussion, that eventually we went ahead with the treatment. By that time my team had changed its attitude entirely and realised that it had been very prejudiced when it first discussed this case at a team meeting.

The initial negative reaction illustrated how easily the principle of a patient's autonomy can be disregarded. 'What if the press got hold of the news that we are treating an HIV-positive patient?' was one loudly voiced objection, as if the rights and wrongs of a person's treatment could be seen in terms of good or bad publicity for the hospital. Others, female members of the staff, said that 'thinking as mothers' they could not allow the unit to bring a child into the world who might die, or whose mother might die. This understandable and emotional response became less easy to justify when it was pointed out that we treated couples with genetic diseases in their families who took identical decisions.

It is presumptuous for doctors to take it upon themselves to decide who would or would not make good parents. This sums up so much of what is wrong with the way we currently deploy some of our medical resources. This is particularly true in the field of infertility which is not a condition perceived as life-threatening. I have no idea whether Sheila with her HIV infection, or indeed any of my patients, would make a good parent. In fact, I am not certain whether I would qualify for that accolade myself. What troubled me then most about this arbitrary process, and still troubles me, is that we impose our values on other people. They are often those who are less articulate, knowledgeable, or well-provided than ourselves and we do so simply because they are suffering from a disease process. No other free member of society is vetted before he or she decides that they want to try for a baby.

Of course people do not have a right to have a child. However, in a society which considers that its citizens should have proper medical care provided for and regulated by the state, those citizens also have a right to fair treatment. That does not always happen in the UK. Whether or not infertile couples get competent, sensitive investigation, whether or not they receive the standard of treatment they have a right to expect, depends on too many irrational, essentially arbitrary and unfair decisions.

Sperm donation

Donors have virtually always been anonymous. This is mostly for the benefit of the donor. Donors do not generally want any responsibility for unknown offspring. The law now requires the donor's name to be recorded in confidential records which must be held by the clinic. This is because it was recognised that children born after donation often feel a need to know about their genetic fathers. The licensing body, the Human Fertilisation and Embryology Authority (HFEA, see page 144), has access to these records. Children have the right to approach the HFEA to get non-identifying information about their genetic parent, such as his walk of life and background.

It is a far from ideal situation. For the donors, who mostly would not be prepared to donate if they had to identify themselves, there is the uncertainty that perhaps the present law could one day be changed. They may enjoy anonymity now but they could find an unexpected child turning up on their doorstep in the future. Hitherto donors have not always been counselled about the implications of what they are doing. They may not fully recognise how their feelings about donating sperm may change in the future. They may not have considered that they will have no idea of whether they have produced any children. Nor may they have given much thought to how a future partner might feel, knowing that somewhere in the background there may be step-children. Research has shown that some donors, long after donation, regret having given semen. They may feel threatened that somewhere they may have offspring whom they do not know and for whom they can take no responsibility.

Keeping a donor register is only of value if recipient families are open about the act of donation. But in many families, DI is kept a closely guarded secret, even from the resulting child. It is my impression that at least two-thirds of parents accepting DI do not inform any close relative, including their child, about the true genetic parentage. This suggests that there is still a deep feeling of misgiving or guilt associated with DI. But although secrecy may seem the least damaging way of dealing with donor insemination, it is a high-risk strategy. Keeping a secret of such magnitude may place great strain on a relationship. Moreover, family secrets have a habit of coming to the surface. A child may possibly discover his true parentage at the worst possible time, perhaps at puberty during an act of serious rebellion, when one parent breaks the news in anger. The secret may surface if the parents split up. If a break does occur, all relationships may be subject to acrimony, and a DI child is at terrible risk. There are other exceptional circumstances when DI children may find that they are not genetically related to their apparent father. A child who is ill with leukaemia and whose only hope of recovery is a transplant from a related donor may find it extraordinary that his 'father' is of totally the wrong tissue type.

Some couples prefer that the donor should be a person they know – usually a close relative, or a particular friend. This, too, is fraught with potential problems. The donor might see his child under parental guidance of which he disapproves. He may find himself feeling very possessive towards the child and attempt to interfere with his or her care in later life. Or an unhealthy bond might develop between mother and donor which threatens the marital relationship. A child may come to perceive that he or she has, in effect, three parents. This could interfere with emotional development, and could cause distress if he or she felt dissatisfied with various parental decisions. These problems could be acute at puberty, when a child most needs a stable nuclear family.

At the time of writing, these issues are very much coming to a head. There is a minority view, from some very responsible people with considerable experience of family counselling, that current arrangements concerning donation do not go far enough. Their view is that it is unacceptable for a child not to know precisely who his or her genetic parents are. The provision of mere non-identifying information, in their view, is inadequate. They want statutory registration of all donors of gametes, so that children can eventually meet any genetic parent, no matter that the parent is no longer involved or responsible for them. They feel that there is evidence to suggest that some children are harmed psychologically because they cannot find out more about their origins. But the problem is, of course, that were identifying information to be insisted upon, the supply of donors might halt completely.

The evidence for the need for identifying information is largely anecdotal. There are no good controlled studies which clearly demonstrate harm. Moreover, most of this anecdotal information is based on the feelings of children who have been adopted and cannot find out more about their parents. I think that it is probable that adopted children are more likely to have these anxieties. After all, they were a baby or a child when handed over for adoption – and this implies a kind of rejection. This seems to be fundamentally different from the child nurtured in his or her mother's womb, but arising from a donated egg or sperm. I seriously doubt whether genetic parentage *per se* is likely to be a very serious issue for most children in this situation, born into a healthy and stable parental relationship. Moreover, the evidence coming out from some long-term studies of children born as a result of sperm donation – particularly those of Dr Golombok of City University – are extremely reassuring.

Whatever the truth about all these issues, it is surely imperative that couples think very carefully about the implications of donor insemination. It is a very personal decision. No one else but the couple concerned can know if it is right for them, but they should certainly seek professional counselling. All registered units offering donor insemination are obliged to offer counselling, so this is relatively easy to get and in most places is given without charge. There are problems associated with donor insemination, but I ought to make it clear that for many couples it is a very fulfilling experience. In many ways it is like adoption, with the advantage that it is much easier to achieve and the child is genetically related to one parent at least.

Women sometimes voice the fear that their partners may not love a child conceived from donated sperm, but this is not a problem in my experience. The male partner becomes deeply involved and shares in the pregnancy and the birth. If the decision is taken mutually and after careful discussion, the man's relationship with the child should be similar to that of fathers with their genetic children. The environment in which we bring our children up is in many ways much more important for their development than the blood relationship. A child will rapidly take on some of the values and outlook of his or her parents, whether or not there is a genetic relationship.

Experts who have studied DI families find little evidence of any emotional or psychological problems. Dr Robert Snowden, Professor of sociology at Exeter University and a leading expert in the field, has many reservations about donor insemination, but agrees that there is no evidence that a child's relationship with a non-genetic father is more likely to break down than one with a genetic father. Dr Margaret Jackson, who pioneered DI in Britain, felt that marriages where donor semen was used were frequently enriched and improved. The very nature of the arrangement involves a degree of commitment that probably very few 'normal' families match.

Even when a donor insemination marriage fails, there is good evidence that the ex-husband's feelings for the children are as strong as they were before and that he continues to want to care for them. It is worth remembering that there are many fathers, genetically related to their children, who treat them appallingly. A genetic relationship is no guarantee of family harmony.

Egg donation

The concerns involved with egg donation are in many ways even greater. Unlike sperm donors, egg donors need to undergo a hefty medical process which is not without physical risk to them. They will need to think about the implications of having offspring they will not know. In addition, because nearly all egg donors have already had children, they have to consider whether it matters that those children will have half brothers or half sisters that they will not know.

The risks and complications involved in egg donation are bound to deter many women from donating eggs. They pose major ethical problems to doctors who allow a woman to run them when she can receive no personal benefit.

A frequently used source of donated eggs at present is probably young women who are undergoing IVF because they themselves are infertile. This is not at all ideal, and many units like our own will only consider using donors of known fertility who are committed to helping an infertile woman. However, many units find it convenient to use surplus eggs from patients whose IVF treatment has left eggs 'surplus to requirements'. So, for example, if patient A produced twenty eggs during an IVF cycle, a few of these eggs would be set aside for fertilisation by sperm from the male partner of patient B, who is awaiting egg donation. There are obvious advantages to this arrangement. These women need to take the drugs concerned for their own treatment and have to have the operation to collect eggs anyway. They are therefore not undergoing any increased physical risk.

Nonetheless, an IVF patient is a very unsatisfactory source of donated eggs. At present there is no way of storing eggs safely. Eggs have to be exposed to sperm within a few hours of being collected from the ovaries. This means that the IVF patient who donates some of her eggs to another woman may find that the recipient of her eggs gets pregnant, but the eggs she retains for her treatment may not fertilise, or, if they do, may not produce viable embryos. In effect, she has gone through an expensive and demanding treatment entirely for the benefit of another individual. I have met women who had this devastating experience and I am convinced that such treatment is unethical.

An alternative source of eggs is to encourage an infertile woman's friends or relatives to become donors. This also raises some very serious issues. We have already seen the emotional and psychological problems that having a related sperm donor can cause a child and its parents later in life. Egg donation is likely to pose similar problems. They may be even greater because of the huge commitment an egg donor will have made. Even if such an act of donation is done with complete love and consent at the time, feelings between the various people involved may well change later. The indebtedness that such a valuable and extraordinary gift produces may well result in different emotions many years afterwards. The donor may well feel extremely possessive about the child that is genetically hers and take more than a dispassionate interest in his or her subsequent well-being.

Some clinics have decided that the only ethically acceptable way of obtaining donor eggs is to collect them when women come into hospital for other gynaecological procedures, such as hysterectomy or sterilisations. This does not solve the ethical problems involved in them having fertility drugs that they would not otherwise have to take. However, it does remove the need for a special anaesthetic or surgical procedure to collect eggs. Those who seek sterilisation are usually quite fertile, hence the request for sterilisation. This fertility is an advantage but the problem with using gynaecological patients is age. Most women having a sterilisation or hysterectomy are close to, or over, 40 years old. At this age, the likelihood is that a very large proportion of abnormal eggs will be produced. It cannot be ethical to transfer defective eggs to an infertile patient, with all the increased risks entailed. An unresolved question is who takes responsibility for the care of the child should he or she be rejected by the bearing mother. Legally there may be no doubt that the bearing mother is fully responsible for any child born to her after egg donation, but the emotional implications for both donor and recipient after such an event are clearly very worrying.

A great difficulty is that as yet there is no firm information about the long-term outcome after egg donation. It is a new field and the oldest child is only thirteen at time of writing. Sperm donation is a poor model because it is so much easier to give sperm than it is to give eggs.

For all these reasons there is a severe shortage of egg donors. Because ovarian failure is common, and because there are an increasing number of older women in their late 30s and early 40s also requesting egg donation, demand for eggs greatly outstrips supply. In our unit, which is not untypical, there is a ratio of around 50 potential recipients for each donor we recruit. But all this may be changed by new approaches. Progress is being made in harvesting eggs from ovarian tissue. It is quite possible to dissect tiny primitive egg-containing follicles from pieces of ovarian tissue without damage to the eggs. Preliminary research (see page 120) shows that it should be possible to mature the eggs retrieved from such tissue so that they can be fertilised.

Surrogacy

Surrogacy arrangements appear to be fraught with moral and legal difficulties. The problem is that because surrogacy arrangements are quite uncommon there is little experience about what kind of nurture might be expected. One problem concerns family relationships. A baby born to a surrogate mother has in reality three parents. This could easily cause considerable confusion for a child, particularly in those cases where the surrogate mother was a friend or relation of the family. The baby may, for various reasons, be rejected by the adopting parents and the surrogate mother may be appalled at the consequences for her natural offspring. She may feel compelled to look after a baby she did not intend to keep. There is also a serious risk that the surrogate mother's attitude to the baby she is carrying may change radically as the pregnancy advances or after the baby has been born. She may decide – as has happened in several well-publicised cases – that she wants to keep the baby, shattering the expectations of the couple who were expecting the child. If a court enforces the surrogacy arrangement, the bearing mother may feel devastated.

If, by chance, the baby is born with a genetic defect, there is a serious danger that it may be rejected by all the parents involved. If the surrogate mother becomes ill during pregnancy, there is the question of who would be responsible for her medical care. And if a surrogate mother doesn't look after her own health during pregnancy, is she to be held responsible for the harmful effects on someone else's genetic child? This has been a real issue in litigation in American courts.

For all these reasons surrogacy arrangements seem to be extremely dangerous. But it is impossible not to feel great sympathy for such couples who often have no other chance to have a baby. Adoption, the only other alternative, is rarely feasible as there are simply too few babies available in most developed countries nowadays.

The attitude of the Government has been to discourage surrogacy although not to ban it. It is a criminal offence for agencies to make surrogacy arrangements on a commercial basis. The surrogate mother herself may receive expenses, although this has often in practice amounted to unofficial payment. In 1997 the Government commissioned a report on the issues raised by surrogacy. The key recommendations of the Brazier report, which was published in 1998, were that payments to surrogate mothers should be restricted by law to genuine and verifiable expenses only; agencies involved in surrogacy arrangements should be registered, and operate according to a Code of Practice; parental orders (giving commissioning parents legal parental responsibility for the child without having to follow adoption procedures) should only be available from the High Court and only in cases where the Code of Practice had been complied with. The likelihood is that these recommendations will eventually receive statutory backing in a new Surrogacy Act.

In practice, there are very few reputable IVF units which are prepared to get entangled in the problems which are raised by surrogacy. Whether attitudes to this difficult, but fortunately uncommon treatment will change remains to be seen.

10
Challenging techniques

Sex selection

For thousands of years humans have sought to determine the sex of their offspring. In ancient civilisations males seemed to have been greatly preferred to females. The worst thing that the Pharaoh could think to do to the Hebrews was to issue decrees for the drowning of all their first-born male children in the Nile, so destroying the providers and the potential soldiers.

The ancients tended to believe that boys were generated from the right side, and girls from the left. Coital position was therefore considered to be an important factor in determining the sex of the fetus. Other factors which at various times have been thought to have an influence include the timing of intercourse during the menstrual cycle, delaying orgasm, changing the amount of salt in the diet or the acidity of the vagina, or taking up a less stressful life-style. There is little evidence that any of these methods worked, but the fact that they were widely used in ancient Egypt, Greece and Rome, and more recently, in many other civilisations all over the world, is an indication of the importance that was attached to being able to determine the sex of a child.

In many societies today, it is still a matter of considerable consequence, and in general there has nearly always been a preference for male children. In some countries with high population growth and low economic development, boys are preferred because they are more likely to become the breadwinners. They are potentially capable of supporting their parents when they are old and infirm. Although the sex ratio between boys and girls is naturally around 106:100 in most parts of the world, in China it is 114:100. There are rumours suggesting the practice of female infanticide which could account for this difference. In parts of India and elsewhere in Asia, ultrasound may also be used in attempts to detect the sex of a baby during pregnancy, and late termination considered if the male genitalia cannot be seen.

The sex of a baby is determined by the sperm fertilising the egg. Sperm carrying a Y chromosome produce males. The Y chromosome is physically smaller than the X chromosome, and there is therefore a minuscule difference in the weight, and possibly size, of male- or female-bearing sperm. Some authors have argued that male sperm swim faster. But in spite of various scientific papers which are occasionally still published on the subject, there is no convincing evidence for the agility or increased speed of Y-bearing sperm. A single sperm weighs less than ten millionths of a gram, and the difference in weight between an X-carrying sperm and a Y-carrying one is probably no more than about three per cent. It is very difficult to measure such a difference accurately, especially when dealing with such a tiny object. None the less, some commercially minded doctors and scientists still attempt to promote methods which claim the successful separation of X- and Y-bearing sperm. These methods all have the object of producing enriched sperm samples for artificial insemination.

The most widely used methods of sperm separation usually involve passing sperm through a high-density fluid, or spinning samples in a centrifuge to isolate those of a particular weight, or a combination of both these methods. Several clinics have now been set up to offer a sex selection service, although there is little independent evidence that their methods actually work. It is notable that these clinics are most common in America, where 'market forces' drive so many of the developments in this area of technology.

Currently, the only proved reliable method of human sex selection is preimplantation genetic diagnosis (PGD), when a cell of an embryo can be analysed for its DNA content. But this is complex, expensive and requires removal of a cell from an embryo – with the possible risk of damage. This is one of the reasons why the HFEA has sanctioned the use of PGD only for those patients at risk of having a baby with a severe disease which is X-linked.

Very soon, however, there will undoubtedly be less expensive and nearly as reliable methods of sex selection. Scientists in Cambridge have enriched sperm samples with X- or Y-bearing sperm by a method known as flow cytometry. This involves placing a fluorescent dye on the X or Y chromosome, after which the sperm can be sorted in a laser beam. The method has been used with cattle sperm with considerable success. There is some question as to whether the fluorescent tagging of the sperm might cause genetic damage, but after these safety concerns have been addressed this approach is likely be used in humans. Incidentally, these safety concerns do not seemed to have carried much weight with at least one clinic in the United States. I see from advertisements on the internet that they are already proclaiming their use of this method. Flow cytometry requires a complex piece of apparatus which needs calibration with considerable expertise but once the sample has been enriched, only insemination is needed. It is therefore bound to be a much cheaper method of sex selection than preimplantation diagnosis with its reliance on IVF.

Eventually, technology like this will open up a huge ethical debate. While it is feasible to regulate sex selection using IVF methods, a more simplified method involving sperm separation and insemination will be almost impossible to police. This will be particularly true in developing countries which have relatively sophisticated technology and where couples are under considerable social pressure to have a child of a specific gender. The lid may be kept on the technique, with difficulty, for a while in Europe but people in Asia may well provide the impetus for the regular use of these treatments.

There are what seem fairly clear arguments against the widespread implementation of sex selection. It could change the balance of the population, probably increasing the ratio of boys to girls. Although this in itself seems highly undesirable, there is little evidence that it would bring about deleterious social pressures. It has been said that sex selection might be likely to increase inequality in society by 'benefiting' the better-off families – an argument which does not seem very convincing. A society filled with males may be more aggressive, but this is also rather doubtful. Should there be a preference for males, it is said that females may find a reduction in their status. But there must be the strong possibility that if males predominated, females would become more 'valuable'. Eventually, there would be pressure, both natural and social, to restore the balance between the sexes. None of these arguments seem to me, therefore, to carry too much weight.

One possibly valid reason for using sex selection might be to allow family balancing. A male child, for example, could be selected in the case of a family which already had three daughters. This, of course, could produce potential harm. In treating a child as a commodity in this way, other siblings may be devalued. Alternatively, the sex-selected child may not reach parental expectations in other ways. But family balancing could be a huge benefit. United Nations predictions demonstrate that within 100 years the world's population (currently around 5.9 billion) will be more than 270 billion if steps are not taken to encourage reduction in the size of families. With two children per family, the prediction is that this increase will only be to a total of around 10.7 billion, a population figure which, though uncomfortable, is certainly likely to be sustainable. Family balancing could be one of a number of advances which could be a way of encouraging a limit on this devastating increase in population.

Cloning

A clone is simply an individual or group of individuals who are genetically identical to one another. Cloning can be a natural phenomenon. Identical twins – occurring when one egg spontaneously splits after fertilisation with a single sperm – are natural clones containing identical genes. Artificial cloning is centuries-old. Plant cloning was a technique well known to the ancient Greeks. MacIntosh apple trees, for example, are all a clone, having been produced from a single mutated plant, and all share identical genes.

Laboratory cloning was first effected by Dr Richard Gurdon in 1968. He transplanted the nucleus of a cell from a tadpole's intestine, into the egg of another frog. The egg had been previously prepared by destroying its own nucleus. Once the new nucleus took over function, the egg divided and grew into a mature frog without any sperm being involved in fertilisation. With the transfer of more nuclei from the same tadpole into more frogs' eggs, many identical frogs could be produced. Cloning in mammals turned out to be much more difficult. Initially, experiments were done using embryonic nuclei because it seemed impossible to use the nucleus of a mature mammal for cloning.

A major breakthrough occurred in 1997 when Dr Ian Wilmut and his colleagues at the Roslin Institute in Scotland announced that they had used the nucleus taken from the mammary tissue of an adult sheep and transferred it to an enucleated egg. The result was Dolly. This announcement caused a wave of the most extraordinary publicity. With it came a huge amount of misinformation, unsubstantiated speculation and simple horror. There was, however, a paucity of rational discussion about the issues involved.

The ability to clone a mammal from an adult cell raised a spectre which still haunts the mind of the public. There was an immediate outcry when Dr Wilmut and his colleagues published their work. Even serious journalists argued that it was now just a matter of time before some rich and powerful man – or worse a political dictator – used this technology to reinvent themselves. Within a few months, an American with a PhD in physics (not obviously ideal credentials for conducting experiments in human reproduction), the appositely named Dr Richard

Seed, announced his attention of setting up a human cloning clinic. He told the world he was intending to make a profit from infertile couples. Since this time, when his publicity campaign appeared on the wane, he has variously announced his intention to clone himself and then to set up a clinic in Korea. Most recently he has announced to the world's media that he has decided, after all, to simply clone his wife. Nobody has thought to ask the question why his announcements should receive any publicity at all.

In spite of the obvious implausibility of his plans, the announcement and a great deal of similar nonsensical and irresponsible publicity surrounding them, served to stoke yet further the widespread fears about the implications of cloning technology. But it is not easy to see a clear ethical objection to cloning a single individual on an isolated basis, not least because twins naturally occur already and their existence presents no obvious ethical problem. Moreover twins are genuinely genetically identical, whilst there are slight variations in a laboratory-made clone. However, the thought of large numbers of clones from a single individual seems very different. But it is doubtful whether there could ever be any practical point in such an exercise, or whether in the foreseeable future multiple copy cloning would be feasible.

There may be a perfectly understandable objection to making many 'carbon copies' of people, but the technology behind cloning is not nearly as threatening as it first appears. Firstly, no individual created by nuclear transfer would be identical to the parent from whom the nucleus was taken. Although nearly all our DNA is held in the nucleus, a much smaller part of it is in the mitochondria – small organelles present in the cytoplasm of the egg. Consequently, the egg as well as the parent nucleus would contribute DNA to that individual. In genetic terms, the individual would be less similar to his or her parent than would identical twins be to each other. Moreover, we are as much a product of our nurture as of our genetic nature. Far too much of our thinking has been based on a deterministic view of genes and genetics. Even twins brought up together are entirely separate individuals, each with their own personality, and interestingly, can sometimes have different genetic disorders. Who knows how a clone of a skin cell of an individual like Adolf Hitler might grow up, given a warm and sustaining environment. He could be loving and gentle, and even contribute greatly to society.

To the public it may seem that reproductive science is moving at great speed, but it must be pointed out that it has taken 30 years of research into cloning to get to the present imperfect state of knowledge. Dr

Wilmut's team at Scotland's Roslin Institute tried repeatedly to complete the first successful cloning from an adult sheep and used hundreds of eggs and embryos in the process. It is important also to remember that the first IVF work was undertaken at the turn of the century, and it took 80 years before the work was applied to humans.

In spite of what has been widely reported, it seems unlikely that the technology presently exists to clone a human being. Numerous embryos would need to be created, and numerous women would need to have an embryo transfer. We are far less fertile than sheep, so a greater proportion of transfers would be needed. But before any transfers in humans, numerous tests on human embryos would be needed to try to ascertain their normal development early in culture.

But even then there would be inadequate evidence that this technique is likely to produce a healthy human clone. The human embryos might look normal and might test normally, but there is every reason to believe that cloning attempts would still be likely to produce an abnormal baby. Hundreds of unsuccessful attempts were needed before Dolly the sheep. Since then a few cloned mice and cows have been lucky to survive. In the early experiments with Dolly, for example, a large number of normal-looking embryos did not survive. More failed to implant. With all cloning experiments there have been repeated miscarriages, and a number of more developed fetuses have died in utero. Fetal death at birth has been common and many of the individuals born after cloning have been overweight at birth or have shown abnormalities of their internal organs. Moreover, the placenta and the membrane surrounding some of these fetuses have been highly abnormal. These unpredictable abnormalities may be caused because cloning upsets the way certain genes express. It is very likely that the growth factors, which control early development, cannot be expressed in normal amounts and consequently there is this loss of life and these abnormalities.

These considerations are sound reasons why it would be very unwise indeed to consider human cloning and I believe that very few doctors or scientists would remotely consider trying it. The chances of abnormality would be excessively high, and leaving aside any ethical consideration, the medical legal consequences to them would be severe indeed. And even where cloning has been successful, there will be grave doubts about an individual's long-term normality. Genetic manipulation of this kind could well produce humans who, though externally normal, might suffer from the rapid development of cancer or accelerated ageing.

Human cloning may pose grave dangers but it would be wrong to be opposed to cloning research. Indeed, there is a great amount of valuable information we can learn. It is important to draw a distinction between the use of cloning for reproduction and cloning to treat disease. Whatever moral and practical reservations may exist concerning reproductive cloning, there is no doubt that therapeutic cloning could have enormous benefits for both human and animal health in the next century. There could be immense clinical value in being able to clone human tissues for medical treatments, and these techniques would be valuable for tissue engineering.

In the very long term, cloning technology might just be used to help men suffering from intractable infertility. Some men cannot produce sperm because their testes are depleted of spermatogonia. It has been suggested that a clone of the father be made and a nucleus placed into the mother's egg. True, for many married couples, this would be ethically much more justifiable than using donor semen from an anonymous donor. Yet making a cloned person might be too risky. But a major refinement of the technology involved could lead to the ability to develop new cells which would effectively replace sperm. Sperm and eggs are different from all other cells in the body in having only one copy of each of the normally paired chromosomes. This state prepares them for fertilisation, so that the egg, when it develops, has paired chromosomes with one copy from the father and one from the mother. Using cloning technologies, it may be possible eventually to remove the nucleus of an adult cell, having manipulated it to lose one set of chromosomes. This nucleus could then be injected as a quasi-sperm into a normal egg, which could then develop like any other embryo, with half its genes derived from the mother and half from the father.

More likely in the nearer future is the use of cloning transgenic animals (see below) kept for medical purposes – for treatments such as organ transplantation. There has been much recent interest in the possibility of using transgenic pigs for heart transplants because of the acute shortage of spare human hearts and other tissues, such as kidneys, livers and heart valves. Once a pig had been genetically engineered to have the appropriate human genes, cloning would provide a convenient way of expanding the herd without loss of the unique genetic make-up needed for medical purposes.

Cloning technology could also help to preserve and breed endangered species. With the potential lack of availability of animals of both sexes in a particular rare species, cloning could be envisaged. Once initial clones had been obtained of a creature threatened with extinction, they could subsequently be allowed to breed naturally so as to encourage normal genetic diversity, which is an important protective mechanism.

With the birth of Dolly, some scientists have claimed that the cloning of cattle could be used to produce whole herds with desirable traits – for example, very good milk yields, or excellent muscle for beef. This may be of value and would seem worth exploration. One serious problem is the lack of genetic diversity in such cloned herds. Given that they would all be genetically similar, they would be susceptible to similar diseases. It is worrying to consider the potential disaster of whole domestic herds being wiped out by being predisposed to a particular infection, or some adverse influence in their environment.

But the immediate importance of cloning is the information these techniques give to the science of biology. What has been forgotten in all this curious debate is that the practice of cloning animals and animal cells, will help the understanding of basic phenomena – for example, the principles of cell regulation. Remarkably, once the adult nucleus is transferred to the egg cell under appropriate conditions, it appears to be totally reprogrammed and effectively starts life from the beginning once again. We have in the nuclei of all our cells, thousands of genes which contribute to the workings of our bodies. Some of these genes are expressed every day in adult life – for example, as you read this page, your brain makes proteins which send the messages across its cells which enable your understanding of what you are reading. You may just have had your supper. Other genes are helping you digest it whilst your muscles, again gene regulated, turn the pages of this book. But other genes in your body have only been expressed once. Those are mostly the genes concerned with development. When you were an embryo, specific growth-controlling and implantation-controlling genes switched on briefly to allow your successful development and survival. The cloned adult nucleus, having been expressing adult genes, suddenly reverts to the beginning of life and starts to ensure that the cloned embryo survives.

This is an extraordinary reversion. It may give us an insight into how the nucleus and its genes can be regulated; how different tissues come to grow from cells which are not differentiated and which have as yet no specific function as bone, muscle or skin, for example. It may be of immense importance for people studying the development of cancers and help us to understand what goes wrong with cells as they grow older and why faults can occur in this process.

Ageing is a key phenomenon; it has puzzled biologists for years yet has critical relevance for the basic understanding of many normal and disease processes. In part, ageing is thought to be produced by deterioration of the mitochondria. These organelles are present in all cells including the egg. The DNA the mitochondria carry is responsible for the metabolic processes and controls some of the ways we use energy sources. It is believed that as we get older, mutations occur in the mitochondrial DNA. These mutations are thought to be associated with the tissue damage associated with ageing. But as we age, changes also occur in the DNA in the nucleus and the telomeres. The tips of the chromosomes become shorter. It is thought that this process may also contribute to ageing. Dolly, therefore, is a fascinating model. She in many ways is the ideal way to explore the phenomena associated with ageing. Is she the age of her adult nucleus, or is she the age of the mitochondria which came packaged inside her egg? It is possible that by deriving the answers to these complex questions, studies on nuclear transfer may go some way to helping understand the ageing process.

Designer babies

As time goes by, we will be able to screen more and more genetic defects through preimplantation diagnosis. But PGD is a complex technique which seems unlikely to be widely applicable because of its cost and its uncertainties. Mankind is inevitably likely to want to explore the potential of going considerably further. Instead of discarding embryos with genetic abnormalities, we may seek to correct those defects by altering our genetic deficiencies.

The study of genetics has led to the greatest advance in medical understanding this century. Probably the most valuable of developments in this field has been the ability to introduce genes into animals – to make transgenics. So-called transgenic technology is providing information which cannot be derived by other means and it is difficult to underestimate its importance in how it is changing medical knowledge. The insertion of a particular gene of interest into a mouse embryo, for example, helps to evaluate what the gene does. By producing mice which, alternatively, have a particular gene missing we can evaluate the interaction of other genes. Gene insertion in animals has started to provide the basis for understanding particular genetic diseases. The mouse can become a model, which can then be treated without risking human life or health. Examining transgenic animals has greatly facilitated our understanding of our early development. It is, for example, playing a key role in learning more about fertility problems and miscarriage. The understanding of the causes of cancer and improvements in therapy are being revolutionised by transgenic work. Coupled with the techniques involved in cloning we may be able produce organs for transplants. But, above all, transgenic technology is the complete model needed to develop gene therapy. This could potentially lead to cures for thousands of genetic disorders and even those diseases which have merely a genetic component.

So far, gene therapy in humans has been limited to inserting genes into somatic cells – cells in tissues such as liver, muscle, nerve cells and the cells which circulate in the bloodstream. But somatic cell therapy only affects the patient treated and not any offspring because the genes inserted do not enter sperm or egg. Germ-line therapy – the insertion of genes into embryos, eggs or sperm so that these genes are inherited – is likely to be feasible in the future. It would be a means of correcting inherited gene defects completely so that future generations would not suffer from the particular disease carried within a family. Ultimately specific gene defects could be permanently eradicated.

There are powerful arguments in favour of germ-line gene therapy. It is a moral obligation for doctors to offer the best treatment possible. Gene therapy treats the disease before it appears, and ensures that future generations will not suffer from it. It does not involve destroying the human embryo but rather protects its 'individuality' or its 'sanctity', depending on your point of view. It could also very likely be the most effective treatment of genetic defects. One limitation of somatic cell gene therapy for diseases such as cystic fibrosis is that by the time gene therapy is started, scar tissue has already formed and there is gross impairment of organ function. So a child with established cystic fibrosis will still be ill, but may not die. He will still suffer from being breathless on exertion, being prone to chest infection, or having retarded growth. Preventing the disease completely, by replacing the defective gene before development, would be medically preferable. Lastly, germ-line therapy will be immensely important to scientific inquiry. There is no doubt that it will enable us to understand much more about how genes enter the embryonic cells and how their expression is controlled.

Where will this technology lead? Once parents are offered the means to correct serious defects in their children, will they not want also to correct less serious ones? Of course, gene therapy becomes one step away from gene enhancement. There are many characteristics that parents, starting a family, might think desirable for their children: resistance against disease, beauty, intellectual power, strength, are just a few of the most obvious examples. Indeed, we already manipulate all of these in our children and young people in varying ways. To give our children disease resistance, we vaccinate them; for beauty, we send them to orthodontists to straighten unsightly teeth; to give them increased intellectual power we send them to the best schools and universities we can; to give them strength we encourage them to exercise and take part in sports.

What is wrong with achieving the same ends more simply, possibly more cheaply and more permanently, by inserting genes and creating 'designer babies'?

Firstly, such treatment may produce an inherited élite, leading to increased tensions in society. One of the greatest moral concerns about all societies are the inequalities which are engendered in them. Genetic engineering could create worse divisions than society has ever experienced before; the risk of a genetic superclass deliberately maintained seems unthinkable at the moment.

Then there would be a risk of children not meeting the expectations of their parents after genetic manipulation, with the resulting fragmentation of family and society. This is already a key issue with regard to screening the fetus during pregnancy. Western society has tended to screen for inherited disorders or handicap. When an abnormality is diagnosed, there is often pressure to have a pregnancy terminated. Opponents of screening claim that it leads to the devaluation of handicapped people and possibly the same would be true in a society regarding genetic enhancement as desirable.

Furthermore, parents' criteria for desirable characteristics are likely to be extremely subjective. Although it may be an advantage in today's society to be tall and blond, in years to come the ideal might be to be short with less back trouble and dark with less of a predisposition to melanomas. It is, in any case, fairly questionable whether most of the qualities generally considered to be desirable could ever be achieved through scientific means. Beauty, intelligence, aggression and so on are not produced by the interaction of one or even a few genes. The genetic component of these traits is extremely complex. To understand just how complex, we can look at the model of disease. Take, for example, diabetes; like height or strength, it has a strong genetic basis. Diabetes is, at one level, a relatively simple disease expression – an inability to regulate sugar levels caused by lack of insulin secretion from cells in the pancreatic gland. This is the essentially basic but invariable mechanism, quite unlike the inherited traits of beauty or intelligence. Yet diabetes is a multigenic disorder: there are at least twenty different genes on several different chromosomes which are likely to predispose a person to developing the disease. Imagine how many different genetic interactions must have to take place for the creation of such poorly defined qualities as beauty or intelligence.

But, above all, the most powerful ethical argument against introducing new genes into human embryos is that the effects of gene insertion are at present unpredictable. In order to inject a gene into a cell, we need to disrupt its basic functions, and that is certainly dangerous. In order for germ-line therapy to work at all, any gene that is therapeutically inserted into the embryo must function normally, providing its usual message to the cell. We would also need to be sure that the gene was incorporated into the DNA at the right point, with appropriate DNA sequences ahead of it, and downstream along the DNA string. Failure to do so could have serious and unpredictable effects. Next, there must be no risk of causing mutations which might affect the individual. It would, for example, be quite unacceptable to cure cystic fibrosis only to find that the 'cured' person has developed leukaemia. Nor should there be any genetic side-effects. The cystic fibrosis might be cured, but other genes cease to function. Or the inserted gene might work for the first year or two of life and then stop expressing.

What do we know about gene insertion in animal models? The most usual model is the mouse because of its availability, and the knowledge we already have about mouse reproduction and mouse genetics. To generate a transgenic mouse, a specific gene, thought to be the cause of a particular human disease, can be injected into the mouse embryo usually immediately after fertilisation. The embryo is then transferred to the fallopian tube or the uterus. If this transgenic mouse develops and is delivered, the effects of the gene can be studied.

Firstly many embryos simply do not implant or become live animals. When they do, most of the time the gene does not take. When it does, the gene may not express its protein product in the normal way. If it does express, expression may not be permanent. The great majority of the time researchers cannot say with certainty what they will be breeding. For example, Dr Carol Readhead and her colleagues at one of the leading laboratories in America, produced transgenic mice which have a problem with myelin production. Although these mice were not seriously ill, their condition provided an important model for the serious human disease multiple sclerosis. The researchers found germ-line insertion to be very dangerous for the embryo. After the gene was inserted, a large number of mouse embryos died, and about twenty per cent fewer embryos than would be expected in the case of normal mouse embryos failed to implant. Among the survivors, the gene was incorporated into the DNA of at most 30 per cent. When the gene expressed, it did so at about only half of full activity. Moreover, the level of expression also fell away after some months. Lastly, in a few of the mice there were mutagenic effects.

Imagine all of this translated into the human. Leaving aside the number of embryos which would die or not implant, there is the unpredictability of everything if a viable pregnancy does form. The cystic fibrosis might be cured consistently in a minor proportion of cases or it might just be less severe. There could be a risk of the full disease returning after a few years. The therapy might cause other essential genes to no longer work, even though it had cured the cystic fibrosis. Then there would be the danger of causing a severe abnormality in the baby.

Undoubtedly, in the far distant future, many of these problems are likely to be solved. But given that preimplantation diagnosis is established, it would be safer and more reliable – with all the drawbacks of its complexity – to continue to use it as the tool against genetic disease. Gene insertion in embryos seems a very long way from any possibility of practical application, and it seems more likely that, when it is finally used, it will be used for therapy rather than to manipulate desired traits. In many decades' time the designer baby may eventually arrive, but conception looks like being very difficult, its gestation would seem to be extremely lengthy, and its birth a moment for an entirely different age.

Tissue engineering

It is possible to grow stem cells from embryos. Stem cells are the basic undifferentiated cells which are capable, under the right circumstances, of growing into particular differentiated tissues. Research over the next decade will give us a much deeper understanding of how cells differentiate. The embryo starts with just a few cells, each of which is totipotential – capable of generating into a complete organism – and one of the great medical advances will be the ability to manipulate embryonic cells so that they grow into just skin, or just muscle, or whatever tissue is needed.

At present, when an individual contracts leukaemia, there is a desperate search to find a compatible bone-marrow donor. Even if one is found, and a bone-marrow graft is successful, there follows a life of immune suppression with unpleasant and expensive drug therapy to ensure that the vital graft is not rejected. In the future it may be possible to treat leukaemia by taking one of the cells from an embryo, and then growing new bone-marrow cells which could be made to be immunologically compatible; consequently there would be no rejection and no need to take immune-suppressive drugs afterwards. This kind of approach, with modification, could be used for skin cells to provide skin banks for burns victims and other patients undergoing plastic surgery for various disfiguring lesions. It could be used to produce nervous tissue cells for transplantation into patients suffering from Parkinson's disease and other degenerative conditions. We could provide banks of muscle cells to treat the muscles of children weakened by various incurable forms of muscular dystrophy.

The embryonic cell that was removed would probably be derived from a blastocyst, though it is possible that with further research, cells from even younger embryos might suffice. Curiously, the biopsy might not mean the destruction of the embryo – the cell could be removed in the same way that preimplantation genetic diagnosis is currently done. This would avoid a potential ethical objection that some people have in that no embryo would be destroyed to produce such tissues. Some researchers have even opined that there might come a time when people engendered from embryos produced by reproductive techniques had a bank of their own embryonic cells held in storage. These would be kept as a kind of insurance for treatments for diseases from which they may suffer later in life.

The artificial womb

In *Brave New World*, Aldous Huxley's wonderfully funny novel, human embryos were kept in vats where they developed into fetuses. Their development could be enhanced by giving them various special food stuffs, so that when they are born they would be most suited to a particular occupation. Embryos could be made identical to each other, so that they could provide a uniform work force. Birth was achieved by a process of decanting.

Aldous Huxley may have predicted IVF and even cloning – but how likely are his ideas about the artificial womb? It is possible to keep the embryos of a rat outside a uterus for short periods of time. However, the embryos have first to be implanted in the uterus to get early nutrition, before they can be removed. This has been used for an experimental model in some of the study in formation of the placenta, and in studies on the mechanisms of action of certain drugs in pregnancy. However, all remaining embryos rapidly become so big that they cannot survive without a proper placenta which is implanted in their mother's uterus. The placenta supplies the oxygen nutrients and other essential compounds which dictate satisfactory growth. One unique aspect of the placenta is that it grows and adapts rapidly to the changing needs of a developing fetus. No man-made machine looks even remotely capable of achieving such a complex function in the foreseeable future. Doctors have managed to make very imperfect artificial organs, such as the kidney machine, and a relatively primitive heart/lung machine. This can keep human patients alive for short periods of time. But the human placenta is in a sense a heart/lung machine, a kidney machine, an artificial liver, and an endocrine gland all rolled into one. Moreover, it grows continuously and its function changes during growth. All these factors suggest that Huxley was fairly wide of the mark.

There is no doubt that an artificial uterus with an artificial placenta would be of huge potential benefit in treating a number of human conditions. First of all, if very premature babies or babies that were miscarried could be rescued by these means, it would be possible to allow them to grow outside the body until they were sufficiently viable to breathe in the open air. But also it would be of huge benefit to women who have the most severe diseases in pregnancy, such as extremely high blood pressure, renal disease and possibly to those who develop cancers during pregnancy.

Recently, there was a report in the newspapers of some work in Japan which suggested they were growing babies outside the womb. In fact the Japanese scientists have been doing some relatively primitive work on sheep. Sheep fetuses, somewhat prematurely born by Caesarean section, were being kept on a kind of life support system in a primitive artificial uterus. The uterus in this case was simply a glass tank filled with salt-containing fluids, and the umbilical cord which carries the blood supply to and from the baby, was being perfused. The best that these scientists could do would be to keep the baby sheep alive for a matter of one to two weeks. There really was extremely little evidence that this technique was truly the development of an artificial placenta or really a way of producing an artificial womb.

But Huxley did spot one thing – he recognised the limitations of cloning technology more that 60 years before we could produce just one animal clone. He saw that techniques for developing clones would be useless unless there were numerous banks of spare wombs in which they could grow. I think it is extremely unlikely that scientists will be able to develop an artificial womb for a very long time to come, if ever. For the time being at least it seems that women will continue to give birth in the old fashioned way and just tolerate the pains of birth and the vagaries of normal sexual reproduction.

Selective reduction of pregnancy

In Britain as we have seen, the number of embryos that may be transferred is controlled. A maximum of three embryos is permitted, but as the reader will understand, we have long advocated the routine transfer of no more than two. Even with the transfer of two embryos a maximum of a twin pregnancy cannot be guaranteed. There have been at least three occasions at The Hammersmith Hospital, where transfer of two embryos resulted in triplets. This is because one of the embryos has split after arrival in the uterus, and formed an identical twin.

But in many countries, there is no limit to the number of embryos that may be transferred. In parts of the United States, for example, some units routinely transfer as many embryos as possible. I have visited one unit in Chicago where it is routine to transfer five embryos if available. In parts of California and parts of the East Coast, I have heard of units transferring as many as eight or nine. These units do this largely because of pressure. They feel that they want to get the highest possible pregnancy rate because this enhances their viability and makes it easier for them to compete with other units. It is in effect 'risking a pregnancy at all costs'. Unfortunately, the costs are born by the unfortunate patient.

Even having twins carries extra risk – statistics show that out of every 23 twin pregnancies, one baby dies. The risk of any twin being handicapped is one in thirteen. High order multiple pregnancy is very serious. There is a much less chance of babies surviving, a much higher risk of miscarriage, a greatly increased chance of fetal abnormality, and these premature babies (as they always are) require a great deal of costly perinatal care. A triplet pregnancy is also extremely disruptive to a family once it is born. The first two years of life are dedicated to feeding and caring for three small infants. This not only destroys any chance of a reasonable social life for many parents, it is tiring and costly. It is not a good start in life for a child.

Fetal reduction of pregnancy has developed against this background. Multiple embryos are transferred, and if there is evidence of more than two or three implantations, selective reduction is offered to the patient. Reduction is normally done using ultrasound control. With an ultrasound probe on the abdomen or in the vagina, a needle is passed into the uterus and thence to a sac containing a pregnancy. With careful positioning, it is possible to introduce the needle directly into the developing embryo, possibly into its heart. There, a number of different compounds may be injected which will result in the embryo dying but which are not toxic to the mother.

It is hoped that most people will have grave reservations about this practice. This is a form of feticide, something which is abhorrent to a great number of people. Psychologically, it can be devastating. The mother knows that she has a number of tiny babies in her womb. A random 'selective' process is going to destroy some of them. I have seen from my own experience that a number of women have bitterly regretted that they undertook the procedure. They mourn the loss of some babies and brood over the arbitrary decision about which ones were sacrificed. They may look at a surviving child and consider the fact that he or she had a brother or sister for whose death they as parents were responsible.

But selective reduction carries with it another serious risk. Trying to remove or kill some of the fetuses can affect the whole pregnancy. It is not uncommon for the pregnancy totally to miscarry after this procedure. It is difficult to imagine anything much worse for an infertile patient: finally to conceive a large number of babies, only to be faced with the decision to have some of them killed, and then in consequence, to lose the whole pregnancy. The feelings of guilt, sadness and depression that follow are very serious. In my view, therefore, selective reduction should never be considered as a kind of routine simply because the doctor was prepared to risk a multiple pregnancy by not taking care. The availability of selective reduction should not dictate the number of embryos transferred, or the dosage of stimulatory drugs given.

Mandy Allwood (see page 170) did not have IVF but underwent routine treatment with drugs to stimulate ovulation. Judging from the press reports, it seems that for various reasons, the treatment and the very early pregnancy may not have been monitored in an ideal fashion. Whatever the situation, Mandy Allwood ended up with an octuplet pregnancy. She was inevitably under huge pressure to have a selective reduction. Certainly, if I had been her doctor I would have recommended it, as it would have at least given some chance of one or two of the babies surviving. As it was, her pregnancy progressed and a selective reduction was not undertaken. Finally, shortly after birth, the babies died, one by one. Such a tragedy must have a deep effect on any man or woman.

It seems mandatory therefore that both routine induction of ovulation and IVF should be conducted with the minimum risk of multiple pregnancy. Deliberately to encourage a high order multiple pregnancy is, I think, irresponsible and probably negligent. However, when a multiple pregnancy of this kind occurs by ill chance, it will continue to seem justifiable to offer selective reduction in every attempt to try and save some human life.

Parthenogenesis

It is possible, under some circumstances, to activate a human egg without actually placing a sperm near it. Certain forms of physical injury will do this, as will a small electrical shock. With activation, the egg may start to divide spontaneously and form a structure which, using routine microscopy, is indistinguishable from a normal embryo. It is for this reason, that in IVF programmes eggs are routinely examined at around eighteen hours, to ensure that there is a genuine embryo, and that any subsequent cleavage is not due to parthenogenesis.

It has been suggested that it might be possible, eventually, to produce a complete human being by parthenogenesis. However, even if the chromosomes were manipulated in some way so that paired chromosomes would be formed, the evidence strongly suggests that lethal genes would prevent further development beyond a few cells. It seems, therefore, that at least for the time being humans will not reproduce like ants, termites or bees. Sexual reproduction may be complicated, but even without the pleasure it brings to many people, I think that it is here to stay for some time.

Amazing revelations, mitochondrial transfusion and old eggs

There was, just recently, a press report suggesting that American physicians were attempting to make old human eggs young! The poor viability of eggs taken from older women is well documented. Moreover, it is known that the ageing process may be due in part to changes or mutations in DNA of the mitochondria (see page 195), the organelles in the substance (cytoplasm) of the egg. They announced therefore a 'breakthrough' in helping older women to successful IVF treatment. Once their eggs had been collected, they transfused them with the cytoplasm taken

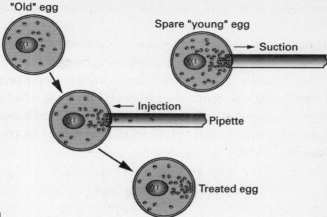

Figure 10.1

from the eggs of younger women (Figure 10.1). By these means, they hoped to give them a kind of royal jelly, or elixir of life.

There are several possible responses to such an experiment. Firstly, it certainly sounds like quite a good idea. It is quite plausible that the reason why 'older' eggs do so badly is because of deterioration in their mitochondrial DNA . There is, after all, no clear evidence of deterioration in the nuclear DNA – and yet 'old' eggs do not function nearly as well.

The second response is highly critical. This piece of 'news' if that is what it is, was published on the front page of a Sunday newspaper. No matter how highly you regard a newspaper – and I, for one, regard this one as a remarkable newspaper – you could hardly call it a leading, peer-reviewed scientific journal. Indeed, a recent trawl through computer records of all relevant scientific journals on electronic databases revealed no published reports at all of this work; several months after the original article. If I am right and this work has not been properly published first, this is surely reprehensible. It raises the criticism that this American clinic is using press publicity to advertise a treatment, in this case for desperate women, without the slightest evidence it works. Yet, regrettably, this kind of thing happens all the time in the field of human reproduction.

Just three weeks before finishing writing this book, a private London clinic announced that it had got the first licence in Britain – that is approval from the HFEA – to freeze human eggs. It announced that they would now be prepared to store eggs from young women for purely social reasons. These women could have their eggs frozen and return much later in life, once they had found their soul-mate, or developed a career. Yet this clinic has not published any research demonstrating that they can freeze eggs successfully, and as we have seen (see page 122) freezing eggs or ovarian tissue requires much more development in humans and animals before we can be sure of its safety, or its efficacy. I find it surprising that a clinic can be allowed by the HFEA to use its name in this way – in what seems to be a frank advertisement.

But, of course, the real cause for concern about mitochondrial transfusion is that human patients – and potentially human babies, if any are born – are being used as guinea pigs. Who knows what the risks of mitochondrial transfusion are? Who knows even if the mitochondria will survive transfusion? Who knows whether there may be the chance of an abnormality in a baby born after such an experiment? The truth is that exhaustive testing should be done in mice eggs first, and then probably other species afterwards. A detailed assessment should be made of whether the mitochondria survive and what the risks of damage to the DNA might be. This is not like an experiment on a cancer victim who is surely going to die unless something is rapidly done. This is a misuse of medical technology and it should be a matter of concern that announcements like these, which happen week after week, are not greeted with more scepticism by the press and with more criticism by those who should be protecting the good name of this controversial and important area of medical practice.

Male pregnancy

IVF techniques could certainly be used to enable men to carry a baby. The human embryo is remarkably invasive and given appropriate circumstances can implant almost anywhere. Ectopic pregnancy is common in women, and pregnancies regularly implant in the fallopian tube. If an embryo goes wandering, it can occasionally implant on the ovary. I have seen ectopics on the bowel, the liver, and in the abdominal cavity. They are dangerous because of the severe risk of massive haemorrhage when they rupture; indeed ectopic pregnancy is one of the commonest causes of women dying in pregnancy.

What is extraordinary, is how difficult it is to have sensible debate about these issues. Just before my seeing the proofs of this book, a leading newspaper got wind of the fact that the book mentions that IVF could certainly be used to enable men to get pregnant. The comments in the media that followed show how inappropriate and unthinking much of the media can be. Dr James Le Fanu writing at the time in *The Daily Telegraph* said 'This type of science fiction serves a double purpose. The first is to impress the public with how brilliant scientists such as Winston must be. The second is to persuade us the allegedly limitless possibilites of science undermine conventional moral values'. It is a pity that Dr Le Fanu appeared not to have reserved his comments until he had read fully what I had written. Had he done so, he might have recognised that his comments are all too typical of those ready to take attitudes about issues involving reproduction. What makes it particularly depressing is that Le Fanu is a qualified medical practitioner and that he backs up his comments by giving what, in my view, are unsustainable reasons as to why male pregnancy is, in his view, impossible.

There is no doubt that men could get pregnant. A man would first need to have doses of female hormones to make him receptive to pregnancy. These could probably be given by mouth – as men hate having injections – and then the embryo could be transferred. It would have to be into a space big enough to accommodate a developing pregnancy and the placenta which goes with it. Ideally, the embryo could be inserted into the abdominal cavity, just under or into the lining – the peritoneum – that surrounds it.

Once implantation had occurred, the man could stop taking hormones because the pregnancy itself would take over. It would secrete sufficient hormone to maintain its own growth and development. No doubt our pregnant man might suffer morning sickness in consequence. He could, without question, cope with the steadily expanding waistline – men are good at this – but might have less patience with the long wait in the antenatal clinic every Tuesday morning. But the real problem would be birth. Delivery would require an open operation to remove the baby, and the real danger would be when the placenta needs removal. This forms such intimate connections with surrounding vessels that its removal would be likely to produce massive haemorrhage. Worse still, implantation might involve other structures in the abdomen, including the bowel and it is possible that part of it would require removal as well. Effectively, our man would suffer all the risks of an advanced and most dangerous form of ectopic pregnancy.

Although this is pretty far-fetched, it does have a serious side to it. Some women are born with a Y chromosome – actually, they are genetically male. They have normal external female genitalia, normal breast development and are quite properly brought up as women, with all the normal female sexual feelings. Because of their curious condition, called testicular feminisation, they do not have a uterus. They are therefore sterile, and not surprisingly, they want children when they marry. Their sterility often becomes the thing which most concerns them, but the risks and dangers in the techniques I have described – of producing an ectopic pregnancy safely – seem insurmountable.

11

Choosing and assessing your treatment

The role of the general practitioner

The point of departure for most couples seeking fertility treatment is their GP. Unfortunately many GPs, and even very many consultant gynaecologists, have too little knowledge of the IVF clinics they recommend. Their experience of IVF is usually minimal, and a couple is probably more likely to get reliable information through their own efforts. Nonetheless, your GP is still the best person to go to for general advice. He can and should have an important role.

There are several excellent infertility organisations which can help couples. The HFEA publishes a *Patients' Guide to DI and IVF Clinics*, which lists all the licensed clinics in the country. Unfortunately the detailed break-down of the success rates which is given in the *Patients' Guide* is always two years out of date. Moreover, these success rates mostly reflect the kind of patients they treat. Clinics which specialise in problem cases will invariably tend to have depressed success rates. The two leading self-help organisations in Britain are CHILD and ISSUE.

To find out the criteria for funding and treatment of their NHS Health Authority couples should contact first their GP and then if necessary their local Community Health Council. They should bear in mind that there will be waiting lists for NHS treatment varying in length according to the particular authority, and that the criteria for treatment may change from year to year. The waiting list is not generally the fault of the clinic – at the moment it is entirely dependent on the programme of treatments that the local health authority has planned to fund. Regrettably, people have virtually no say over which NHS clinic they are referred to. They may have to accept what they are offered.

People are entitled to seek treatment as private patients and NHS patients at the same time, as long as they have a separate referral letter from their GP. But some District Health Authorities may withhold NHS treatment from patients who have already had private treatment. This is something that you may need to check locally.

Choosing a clinic

The first thing that must be said is that British IVF is of a very high standard. Most clinics are honest, caring and competent. Over the last years there have been remarkable improvements in reproductive medicine. There is a highly polished training programme in this relatively young speciality, and there are more excellent doctors practising in it than ever before. This was not always the case, hitherto. The HFEA has also played its part. Whatever the pains and limitations of regulation, the HFEA has consistently helped make improvements in the information given to patients and the standard of treatment and counselling they receive. Now perhaps it is the NHS which has the most work to do. For too long it has not regarded these treatments as sufficiently important.

At the present time NHS patients have very little or no choice about which IVF unit they attend. This has been restricted by the various local purchasing arrangements organised by health authorities. If you are lucky enough to a) have funding and b) have a choice, you should consider a number of points. These considerations are absolutely relevant to those people considering private treatment, too. Here are some of them:

- Did you like and feel confident with the clinic's team of doctors and nurses? Did they seem like a team? If so, the chance of good communication, so vital to feeling happy about the treatment, is likely to be adequate.
- Do patients regularly see a doctor rather than a member of the paramedical staff? Do they see the same individuals during treatment? Good units try to ensure good continuity of care and communication because so many patients are otherwise confused by conflicting information.
- Does the clinic carry out adequate tests to establish a clear diagnosis before treatment? This may seem beyond the competence of a lay person to decide, but it is fairly simple to find out if the doctors take a uterine X-ray (hysterosalpingogram or HSG) when needed, or personally examine X-rays taken earlier at another hospital. If you merely ask, 'Do you do the necessary tests?' the clinic may simply say yes. So you could ask, for example, specific questions about what tests the clinic finds are important in unexplained infertility. The list in

Chapter 2 of this book may be helpful to you in this respect. Does the clinic also do other key tests, such as hormone tests at the beginning of the menstrual cycle, detailed scans, proper sperm function tests, before committing a patient to IVF? Beware of the clinic which only offers you the expensive lucrative tests – such as laparoscopy – especially if they offer them first.

- Does the clinic have an independent counsellor offering a free service? It is important that patients should have the opportunity to talk to someone who has not been involved in their treatment and can therefore offer them objective advice on what might be best for them. This counsellor should not be involved in giving clinical information, but rather helping you to find out how you feel about what is happening to you.

- Does the clinic provide a comprehensive range of fertility treatments? Clinics which offer IVF as their chief or only treatment tend to offer it to the exclusion of other treatments. This is convenient for them, but may not be in the best interests of their patients.

- How thoroughly is the treatment cycle monitored? Generally, clinics which do regular hormone tests get better results and may have fewer complications; they also have a better idea of what went wrong if the treatment fails.

- Does the clinic have a fixed drugs regime for stimulating women to produce eggs, or does it tailor the treatment to suit the body and circumstances of the particular individual?

- Are careful and repeated assessments of sperm quality made before IVF treatment is undertaken? A good unit will have a set of precisely worked-out values for sperm quality, and will cancel an attempt if it thinks that there is no chance of fertilisation.

- Is it possible to make weekend appointments if you have a problem? Are they able to offer egg collections and inseminations on most days of the week? If they can only do these treatments two or three times a week, your success may well be jeopardised.

- Is there a choice of local or general anaesthesia and is an anaesthetist invariably present during egg collection to ensure the patient's safety?

- Do their embryologists examine the eggs eighteen hours after mixing them with sperm? This is essential to ensure that a dividing egg has really fertilised (see page 10).

- How many embryos do they routinely put back into the uterus? Clinics putting mostly three back, particularly in women under 35, are probably taking risks in attempts to improve their pregnancy rate.

These data can be checked in the *Patients' Guide* and the triplet rate, which is also recorded, can be revealing. A good clinic should be getting no more than two or three sets of triplets per thousand IVF cycles.

- How much does the clinic charge? If it charges much more than other clinics – the average cost in a private clinic of an IVF cycle, excluding drugs, is around £1,500–£2,000, they may be overcharging. On the other hand, if they are charging much less than say £1,200 they are almost certainly not offering the most effective treatment. Costs should be inclusive apart from drugs; be wary of clinics that charge huge hidden costs – for example for extra ultrasound examinations, extra consultations, and pregnancy tests.

- If the treatment fails, will you be able to see the director of the clinic personally? In good clinics, the director or somebody who holds the equivalent of an NHS consultant post should be available (by appointment) to see couples who have failed their treatment cycle. He or she should be able to discuss the progress of the cycle, working out what, if anything, went wrong, where improvements might be made and to advise on whether a further IVF attempt should be made or if other treatment should be considered.

Assessing the *Patients' Guide*

The Patients' Guide to DI and IVF Clinics (most recent edition December 1998) lists the results of each clinic. There are some important things to understand about these results. In general they are not a particularly good way of choosing where to go. To help understanding, table 10.1 gives a fictitious clinic's results – with the boxes laid out as in the HFEA guide.

The first thing to understand is that these results are unadjusted and comparison of the results between clinics is almost meaningless. Even if one clinic reports a success rate of around 27 per cent and another say only ten per cent, there is statistically no difference between them. This has been shown by careful analysis by competent statisticians to be so. The results in any clinic depend primarily on the kind of patient they are treating – their age, their cause of infertility, the length of time they have been trying, the number of cycles with ICSI, the number of cycles of IVF they have already failed and the ability of their ovaries to respond to drugs. These factors vary hugely from clinic to clinic and between different areas of cities. Remember too, that data collection and publication take a long time and the figures reported are on average over two years out of date.

Box 1. This simply shows the address of the clinic, its phone number and what the HFEA has licensed it to do. Note that GIFT is not a licensed procedure but will be mentioned in Box 1 if the clinic is licensed to use GIFT and donor eggs or sperm.

Box 2. This gives the raw, uncorrected data for IVF, including IVF with ICSI. In the first line, the percentage live birth per embryo transfer is shown, the next line per egg collection and the third line per cycle started. In general the differences between the first two figures should not be more than about two per cent – if they are, it could suggest sub-standard laboratory work. The difference between lines two and three is not very meaningful – but a gap of around three per cent or more argues that the clinic is cancelling cycles before egg collection if it feels that there is a poor chance of success. In most cases, this will be to try to save its patients money because cycles stopped before egg collection are generally charged at a small fraction of the total cost.

Box 3. This is the most informative box and may repay analysis:
1. Line 1 is the number of patients treated, line 2 the number of cycles. Clinics with more than around 600 cycles are large clinics and are generally a bit more successful. They should have enough data to be able to provide a computerised breakdown of your chance of success for a particular circumstance – based on results from other patients under their care. Line 3 is relatively meaningless.
2. Line 4 is the number of ICSI cycles. The higher the percentage, the better the overall success rate in Box 2 should be. Clinics with many ICSI cycles (say more than 25–30 per cent) and a lower overall success may not be doing so well.
3. Line 5 is the percentage of cycles with more than two embryos transferred. Clinics with a high percentage may well be taking risks in attempts to improve their pregnancy rate.
4. Line 6. The percentage of abandoned cycles. In general, clinics with a low rate may generally be dealing with the easiest patients to treat, or may be not prepared to abandon cycles to save their patients an unnecessary egg collection.

Box 4. This simply gives the number of donor cycles. If you are seeking egg donation you may find it best to seek one of the clinics with a high figure – as they are more likely to be able to find a suitable donor.

Box 5. Deals with frozen embryo transfers. The percentage is not recorded here so you have to work it out for yourself; anything over ten per cent is respectable and suggests competent laboratory work.

Box 6. Deals with results of DI and may reflect on the quality of IUI that that clinic does as well. Anything above ten per cent would be considered respectable.

Centre 0303
St Jude's Hospital Assisted Conception Unit

In Vitro Fertilisation Treatments

Non-adjusted live birth rates derived from stimulated fresh embryo IVF, including ICSI*

Non-adjusted live birth rate *Per embryo transfer*	18.2%
Non-adjusted live birth rate ***Per egg collection***	**17.9%**
Non-adjusted live birth rate *Per treatement cycle started*	15.0%

*excluding frozen embryo transfers, unstimulated treatments and treatments
  with donated eggs and embryos*

Results for all IVF Treatments

Patients treated	566
Total treatment cycles	1180
Stimulated treatment cycles	978
Treatments using ICSI	198 (16.8%)
Cycles where two embryos transferred	156 (13.2%)
Abandoned treatment cycles	73 (6.1%)
Singleton births	106
Twin births	58
Triplets	11

Treatments with donated eggs or embryos

Cycles with donated eggs	12
Cycles with donated embryos	8
Number of live births	2

Frozen embryo transfers

Number of frozen embryo transfers	70
Number of live births	11

Donor Insemination Treatments (excluding GIFT)

Non-adjusted live birth rate *per treatment cycle started*	**10.9%**

All Licensed DI Treatments

Patients treated	98
Treatment cycles	128
Stimulated treatment cycles	52
Singleton births	11
Twin births	2
Triplet births	1

Gamete Intra Fallopian Transfer (donor gametes only)

Number of GIFT treatment cycles	0

Should you try IVF again?

Probably the most important job that I do in my own clinic is to see as many as I can who have failed an IVF treatment cycle. Invariably, the couples who come to see me after failure basically ask one question. Should I try again? This is probably the most complicated question in the whole of reproductive medicine and it is very difficult to give advice.

The first thing to remember is that, most of the time, failure is simply a matter of statistical probability. IVF only has around a one in five chance of success. If you had placed your money on a horse at five to one against and it had not won, you would not have thought that there was anything abnormal about it. So much of the time, going through a repeated cycle is just about increasing the odds a little in your favour.

Other times there may be assessments you need to make. You cannot always expect your doctor to tell what you should do because most good doctors will feel quite presumptuous in telling a patient either to continue, or to stop. So here is a list of some questions, and points that may be valuable in trying to come to this most difficult of all decisions.

How did you both feel about the treatment?

For some people, going through IVF is a harrowing experience, one that they do not really wish to repeat. For others, it is a great deal easier than they expected and they often find that there is much that is positive about it. I have no doubt, therefore, that one of the questions that should be top of this list, is your own assessment of whether you found going through treatment depressing and difficult. If you did, you should certainly think very seriously before trying again, and I would strongly advise talking to a third person.

Nearly all good clinics offer in-house counselling with a professional counsellor who has great expertise in helping people to pinpoint what their feelings really are. This is a subject with which they deal on a daily basis and they are a most valuable resource when trying to arrive at decisions concerning repeated treatment. Far too often, people underestimate the value of good counselling sessions. No counsellor will be able to tell you what to do, but will enable you to focus on the crucial aspects of how you feel, and will help you to make your own mature judgements about further treatment.

Can I afford it?

I think that this is a question which is possibly not asked often enough. *In vitro* fertilisation is an expensive business. Moreover, subsequent treatment cycles are often more expensive because as a woman gets older, she tends to need more drugs to stimulate the ovaries. It is quite common for the amount of gonadotrophin rapidly to increase with successive treatment cycles, and the drug costs may spiral.

I think there has to be a very serious assessment about whether or not it might be better to spend your money in other ways. This, I think, is particularly true for those patients who already have one child. Sometimes it may be better to consider spending the money on your existing family, rather than in forlorn hope to try to increase it.

What does the computer say?

More and more of the larger clinics now have a considerable database on which are recorded a large number of treatment cycle attempts. Many of them use the excellent database designed by Dr Hossam Abdulla and his team at the Lister Hospital in London. Clinics that are doing over five or six hundred cycles a year, and have been in existence for a long time, will have an increasingly broadened experience of various medical conditions which impinge on the chances of success or failure of an IVF cycle.

All good units keep excellent computer records and more and more of them are able to give an assessment of the mathematical chances of success or failure given another treatment cycle. It is not unreasonable to ask, for example, 'Given a patient of my age, with tubal disease, one previous pregnancy, and two failed attempts at IVF, what are the chances if I undertake a third cycle?' Clearly to answer this kind of question accurately from the computer a unit needs a very large database – there are four variables in it – age, tubal damage, previous pregnancy, and considering a third cycle attempt. But those that have several thousand patients may well be able to provide some valuable insights into the difficult decision you are about to take. Obviously, the computer will not answer everything. For some people, a three per cent chance is worth taking. For others, a fifteen per cent chance is not worth consideration.

Are there genetic factors?

Some women clearly have a family history of an earlier than average menopause. It is worth finding out how old your mother was when you were born and how old she was when your brothers and sisters were born. The age when your mother stopped having periods may also be a helpful indication. Women whose mothers tended to have an early menopause, may in turn themselves have an earlier than average menopause. Under these circumstances it may be worth trying treatment as soon as possible, then giving up, particularly if there is a poor response to superovulation.

Assessment of the previous treatment cycles

A visit to the clinic for a troubleshooting session after failed IVF needs thorough perusal of your medical and laboratory records. There are a number of pointers which will help tell you whether or not a further treatment has a good or bad prognosis.

Response to stimulation

Patients who require only a small amount of gonadotrophin, perhaps less than 30 ampoules, are likely to have a much better chance of success should they repeat a treatment cycle. In general, this also tends to be true of patients with a tendency to hyperstimulation. Conversely, those women who need massive doses of drugs to induce ovulation are likely to have a much poorer chance with successive attempts. If for example, you required 80 or more ampoules of gonadotrophin to get to egg collection last time, you do need to think very seriously about whether it is worth going for another treatment cycle. The chances are very strong that you will be likely to need more gonadotrophin and it is also likely that your chance of a pregnancy will be even worse than it was with the last treatment.

Egg numbers

People yielding a reasonably large number of eggs, say more than seven or eight, have a statistically better chance of success in another treatment cycle, than those that have yielded five or less. The number of eggs collected after stimulation is partly dependent on age. Most clinics will be able to tell you the average numbers of eggs they expect from a given age. If you are much below this average, it is an indication that another treatment cycle is less likely to be successful. For example, a woman of 35 should produce an average of around ten eggs. A woman of 38 who is producing less than four eggs has a very poor chance indeed.

If you have had several treatment cycles, then adding up the total number of eggs you have produced is also helpful. Moreover, if the number of eggs is decreasing with each attempt, this is further evidence of a reduced chance of success.

Oestrogen levels

Most good units take several blood samples to measure the oestrogen values during an IVF treatment cycle. These are a useful indication of how well the ovary has responded and what its chance is of responding in another cycle. Some units pay particular attention to the peak oestrogen value, that is the highest level achieved, usually just before the egg collection. Women who produce low levels, say below 2,500 pmols per litre, are likely to have a much poorer chance of success in a further treatment cycle. As successive treatment cycles are done, the ovaries tend to become increasingly refractive – that is to say, they tend to fail to respond. Poor response in general carries a poor prognosis for future treatments. Like egg numbers, this too is to some extent age related. Nevertheless, a woman of 42 or 43 who produces peak oestrogen levels of more than 5,000 pmols per litre is likely to have a much better chance of IVF success should she try again.

Fertilisation rate

People who are producing poor quality eggs will tend to have a low fertilisation rate. The average, not using ICSI, should be around 60 per cent. Patients who are falling well below this level in the presence of normal sperm are likely to be producing eggs which may not give rise to a good embryo. Very poor fertilisation rates, if they are repeatedly seen over several cycles, are a good indication of poor prognosis. Some units try to get round this problem by forcing fertilisation with ICSI. I think it is an open question whether or not ICSI is really of much benefit in these circumstances. On the whole, you cannot force a bad egg to become a good embryo simply by injecting a sperm into it.

Spare embryos

Your previous treatment cycle may have generated a number of spare embryos. Sometimes these will of course have been frozen. Other times they will have been grown for a while in culture. The observations made on the spare embryos' culture are extremely valuable. If, for example, a number of these embryos grew to the blastocyst stage, this is pretty good evidence that you are producing better than average embryos. Clinics often tell patients that their embryos 'look good down the microscope'. As I have said earlier it is impossible to tell whether an embryo is good or bad merely by looking at it. But a number of units are doing research on spare embryos, and it is your prerogative to have access to these results. The research embryologist's observations on these embryos may give some real clues as to how good the embryos are that you are capable of producing.

Preimplantation genetic diagnosis

Some units are now doing dynamic tests on embryos, which tell us more about the chromosomes within them, and the chemical the embryos are producing. These tests are going to be increasingly valuable when used on spare embryos. With further research and development, they may also give a helpful clue as to the quality of the embryos that have been transferred. In due course, preimplantation genetic diagnosis testing may well be available for the embryos that have actually been transferred. This will be particularly useful for some women with repeated failure, and women in the older age group. This is something that might be worth considering when trying to work out where to go for a further treatment.

Failed pregnancy

If a previous IVF cycle has ended with a failed pregnancy even if it has been an ectopic, a miscarriage, or merely a biochemical pregnancy with a slightly raised level of HCG in the bloodstream, the prognosis is better for another attempt at treatment. Women who have had a child in the last four or five years, are also in a better category and it may be worth their while persisting with further IVF attempts. It does not matter whether the pregnancy was conceived spontaneously, or by IVF. The prognosis is still improved when compared with IVF in women who have never conceived at all.

Tests before another treatment cycle

FSH levels

Blood levels of FSH tends to rise as the ovaries fail. A test of FSH should be done between the fifth to the ninth day of an unstimulated cycle in the assessment of whether to repeat IVF attempts. If this level is much over 10 international units, then the chances of IVF working, if repeated, are reduced. Above 15 international units and the chances of success are very poor indeed. High levels indicate that the ovaries are failing and are unlikely to respond to stimulation. It is virtually never worth considering IVF if the level is over 20.

Sadly, once the FSH level has been found to be raised – even if the level returns to normal values – the prognosis is still exceptionally bad.

Ultrasound assessment

FSH levels are not the only indication of a likely poor response from the ovaries. It may be useful to have an ultrasound of the ovaries before repeating IVF. Apart from excluding cysts which may occur following stimulation, assessment of the total volume of each ovary has been quite valuable in our clinical experience. Patients with very small ovaries, say below a volume of three millilitres, are likely to have a poor response if ovulatory drugs are repeated.

The uterus

Sometimes, regrettably, IVF units forget to assess the uterus. There is no question that this should be done before any fertility treatments. Nevertheless, if it has not been done – or not been done within the last four years or so – I would strongly recommend getting accurate information about the state of the uterine cavity and its surrounding muscle. Although units frequently offer a hysteroscopy, a better test is undoubtedly the hysterosalpingogram (HSG). It is also cheaper. Providing this is done properly in a good unit with good imaging technique, it is not painful. It can give the most valuable information about the condition of the uterine cavity. Very frequently there will be defects in the cavity which are correctable before considering another IVF attempt, or fibroids which should be removed.

Chromosome assessment

A number of men and women have unexpected chromosome problems which may give rise to their infertility, and which have not been diagnosed. It is certainly worth getting blood tests from both partners to evaluate this if the cause of failure remains puzzling. These tests are not cheap, unfortunately. Ideally, a large number of white cells from the blood should be examined and not just the routine one or two. This is because sometimes people may be 'mosaic'. That is to say, they have some cells in their body which have a normal chromosome complement and others which do not. Even patients with a mosaic may have a slightly higher risk of producing abnormal embryos and a greater chance of infertility or miscarriage. If this is the problem, currently there is only a limited amount that can be done. A few units are offering preimplantation genetic diagnosis, but the assessment of most of these chromosome disorders is still difficult at the present time.

What you can do before another treatment

Weight loss

There is no question that moderate obesity (or worse) is a significant reason for all assisted conception treatments to fail. I would strongly advise anybody to try to get to as close to a normal weight as possible before undertaking them. Nonetheless, if you are still overweight and have failed a treatment cycle, it really is in your interest to do something about it. This will almost certainly mean not only diet, but a degree of regular exercise. However, it is probably not wise to go through an IVF treatment cycle whilst starving. It is best to wait until one's body weight is in equilibrium.

General fitness

There is not much evidence one way or another as to whether general fitness makes much difference. However, there is some evidence that smoking, and very excessive alcohol, might reduce the chances of getting normal eggs. They certainly reduce the chances of getting normal sperm. Whilst the evidence is poor that these factors make much different to the eggs, it probably does not make much sense to go through these treatments in a toxic state.

Alternative treatments

The 'short protocol'

As women get older, they respond less well to gonadotrophins. Also, many women do not respond particularly well to the drugs which suppress pituitary function, like Buserelin. This effect tends to be more pronounced with increasing age. If you had a poor response to stimulation last time and are in the older age group, it might be worth discussing the short protocol (sometimes referred to as the 'flare-up protocol') with your doctor. With these treatments, Buserelin or similar drugs are only given for a very short time, and gonadotrophins are started before the FSH is suppressed. Some units have had a better success rate with this protocol in older women, or in those with a poor response to superovulation. Other units have not, and it is worth discussing their findings very carefully with them.

Hydrosalpinx (water on a fallopian tube)

It is clear from various statistics that if you have tubal disease your chances on the whole are less good. There is loose evidence that patients with blocked fallopian tubes containing fluid do less well than patients who have normal tubes, or patients with damaged tubes which do not contain fluid. Some units, including our own, have had an increasing number of pregnancies after repeat IVF having first dealt with hydrosalpinges. One way of approaching this is to undertake a laparoscopy and to remove the offending blocked swollen tube. Another strategy is to clip the tube off where it joins the uterus using the kind of clips which are normally applied during sterilisation procedures. Once this has been done, any infected fluid inside the fallopian tube cannot then drain into the uterine cavity. It is thought that this may decrease the chance of compromising the uterine environment. There is no clear statistically proved evidence that treatment of hydrosalpinges makes a substantial difference but there is quite good anecdotal evidence that it may be worth trying in some women.

Donor eggs

There is no question that particularly for women who have a poor response to superovulation, or for those that produce very poor eggs that do not fertilise well, an egg donor could be the answer. This is a major decision to take, and should certainly be preceded by thorough counselling. It is worth emphasising that there are far more women seeking a donor egg than there are numbers of donors prepared to give up their eggs. One hopes that in the future, with improvements in technology, donor eggs may become much more available. In my view, you should not attempt using donor eggs if there is any reasonable chance that your ovaries can produce your own. Sometimes, it is my impression that some clinics tend to offer donor treatment too early, before all else has been explored.

Treatment of tubal disease

A very large number of patients come to us with tubal damage. Many of them have had repeated attempts at IVF which have failed, but they have never had any operation on their fallopian tubes. There is no doubt that in the right cases, providing that patients are carefully investigated and selected, the results of tubal surgery are undoubtedly better than the results of IVF. This is particularly the case if the tubal surgery is done with proper microsurgery and an expert surgeon with good experience. At The Hammersmith Hospital in the last two years, I have operated on seventeen patients who between them have failed no fewer than 86 treatment cycles of IVF. Eight of these patients have now had a pregnancy after tubal surgery. Two of them had already had five IVF attempts each. Surgical correction is also valuable for those women with problems in the uterus. It makes no sense to go through repeated treatment failures when there are fibroids distorting the uterus. Their surgical treatment is strongly recommended in such circumstances, particularly if the uterine cavity is distorted.

It is worth considering that many women just do not respond very well to superovulatory drugs. It is these women who may well do much better by tubal surgery, because it is a gentler treatment. It is interesting, that a number of the patients we have treated successfully with tubal microsurgery, were very poor responders when given drugs to stimulate ovulation.

When to give up treatment?

Clearly, it is not sensible to continue to have IVF treatment against all odds. Many women feel that they wish to gamble in this way, but they may be betting with their health and with their feeling of well-being. If you have been through IVF more than once or twice, and have had consistent testing then you should know that you have left no reasonable stone unturned. This in itself should be an important consideration. You should not be planning to have endless repeated treatment cycles, unless the portents clearly indicate some reasonable chance of success.

Whilst you are a patient, your situation remains unresolved. Please do not end up 'enjoying being a patient' – that is getting psychological support from treatment and avoiding the inevitable. All of us, at sometime in our lives have to lose something we most value. When we lose a parent for example, we have to mourn, but we do get over this terrible blow. Giving up infertility treatment is not unlike this in many ways. Taking the decision to stop, taking the decision to grow through a period of mourning, can be a positive experience. Normal people, though they feel desperate at the time, come out of this feeling much better and stronger. Once you have given up infertility treatment, your whole life can be resolved and you can get on with the other valuable things within it.

It is worth bearing in mind that during the course of this book, I have written many things which are depressing about infertility treatment. What I have not said much is that it can be an enriching experience. This may sound strange, but so many couples find that it has strengthened their relationship and that it has enabled them to deal with other problems in a much more sensible and focused way. Infertile people, if they are not careful, can allow their treatment to destroy their well-being and to destroy the things and relationships they most value. It is unwise to let this happen to you. It is worth recognising that you have gone through definitive treatment and may now need to close the door.

Glossary

Adenomyosis The condition which is caused by pockets of endo-metrium – uterine lining – growing in the muscle wall of the uterus. When the resultant scarring is severe, it may cause painful periods, irregular cycles, and infertility.

Adhesiolysis Division of adhesions using a laparoscope or via an open operation.

Adjuvant A compound or process which improves a treatment.

Amniocentesis A method for detecting abnormalities of the fetus during pregnancy. Samples of fluid are drawn off using a fine needle inserted into the womb and analysed for chromosome or chemical abnormalities. It is a common method for diagnosing Down's syndrome.

Anastomosis Joining two tubes by their cut ends.

Antibodies Formed as part of the body's defence system against foreign invasion, for example bacteria. Sperm antibodies are an example of what happens when the system 'goes wrong'. The antibodies detect sperm as foreign protein and they fail to function.

Asherman's syndrome Scarring and adhesion formation inside the uterine cavity, often causing infrequent or scanty menstruation and infertility.

Beta-thalassaemia A severe inherited form of anaemia caused because the haemoglobin molecule does not form normally.

Biopsy The surgical removal of a small piece of tissue for analysis.

Blastocyst Stage of embryonic development at around five days, just before implantation into the womb. At this stage the embryo is a fraction of a millimetre across and comprises something over 100 cells.

Buserelin Drug used to reduce the activity of the pituitary gland in the brain. Often administered by sniffing. Its use for two or three weeks prevents the ovary from producing its own follicles or hormones without external stimulation by fertility drugs. The effect is reversible within hours of stopping Buserelin.

Catheter   Fine tubing mostly used to transfer embryos, eggs or sperm to the uterus, fallopian tubes or vagina.

Chromosomes   The paired structures on which the genes are located. One of the pairs is inherited from the father, the other from the mother. Each human cell contains 23 pairs of chromosomes.

Chorion villus sampling   A method of detecting abnormalities of the fetus during pregnancy. Because it involves taking cells from the developing placenta, it carries a slightly increased risk of miscarriage.

Clomiphene   The common fertility pill, taken in the first part of the menstrual cycle. It helps ovulation by stimulating FSH production.

Cornu   The part of the uterus where it joins the tube.

Cryopreservation   Storage at temperatures well below freezing point – usually in liquid nitrogen at around minus 200° Celsius.

Cystic fibrosis   An inherited disorder which affects roughly 1 in 1600 individuals in the population. Sufferers are often underweight, have frequent severe chest infections, and digestive problems.

Deletion   A disorder caused by a missing piece of DNA in a gene, or an entire missing chromosome.

DNA   The chemical blueprint contained in the chromosomes, of which genes are made.

Dominant gene defect   A disorder which is caused when one parent has a particular misprint in a dominant gene. Any child born from such parents will have 1:2 chance of being affected by the disorder.

Down's syndrome   This genetic condition is caused by three copies (or trisomy) (instead of a pair) of chromosome 21. It leads to mental retardation.

Duchenne muscular dystrophy   A fatal genetic defect. It is sex-linked, affecting only boys. It causes progressive muscle-wasting, necessitating life in a wheelchair.

Ectopic pregnancy   Pregnancy outside the uterus – usually in the fallopian tube – which can occur in any woman with tubal damage, even after IVF.

Endometrium   The lining of the womb, shed during menstruation.

Endometriosis   Abnormal deposits of womb lining (endometrium) outside the womb, usually in organs nearby. It may cause some internal bleeding and pain is common, especially during periods.

Epididymis   The fine coiled tubing which conducts sperm from the testis to the vas deferens.

Falloscopy   Examination of the fallopian tube by inserting a very fine telescope through its inner (uterine) end.

Fibroid   A benign tumour of the uterus more common in women over the age of 38 years.

Fimbria   End of the fallopian tube near the ovary.

Follicle   The cystic structure in which an egg develops in the ovary.

Follicle stimulating hormone (FSH)   Hormone produced by the pituitary gland, causing the ovary to produce follicles and eggs. In men, FSH stimulates spermatogenesis (q.v.)

Fructose   A sugar required as an energy source for sperm, produced by the seminal vesicles – the storage area connected to the ducts coming from the testicles.

Gamete intrafallopian transfer (GIFT)   The treatment by which eggs are removed from the ovary, mixed with sperm and then returned to a fallopian tube before fertilisation.

Gene   An active part of the DNA responsible for making a particular protein.

Genome   The complete sequence of the DNA in a species. A species is, in essence, defined by its genome.

Germ-line gene therapy   Introducing new genes into a sperm, egg or embryo with the idea of curing a genetic defect.

Gonadotrophins   Hormones – LH or FSH – produced by the pituitary gland which stimulate the testes or ovaries.

Human chorionic gonadotrophin (HCG)   A hormone which mimics the action of LH, encouraging the ovary to develop follicles to ovulate.

Human Fertilisation and Embryology Authority (HFEA)   The government regulatory authority set up under the Human Fertilisation and Embryology Act 1990.

Huntingdon's chorea   A severe neurological disorder caused by a dominant gene. The disease usually starts in middle age and is characterised by uncontrolled writhing movements and mental changes.

Hydrosalpinx   A collection of watery fluid in a blocked fallopian tube.

Hyperstimulation   Over-vigorous response of the ovary to fertility drugs, causing swelling of the ovary and discomfort. Sometimes called **Ovarian hyperstimulation syndrome (OHSS)** which, when severe, can cause severe disturbance requiring hospital admission.

Hysterosalpingogram (HSG)   The X-ray examination which outlines the uterine cavity and tubes by injection of a radio-opaque dye.

Hysteroscopy   Telescope inspection of the inside of the uterine cavity.

Immotile   Not moving.

Intracytoplasmic sperm injection (ICSI)   Sperm injection directly into the egg to assist fertilisation.

Intrauterine insemination (IUI)   Freshly produced semen is washed and filtered in the laboratory and then immediately injected into the uterine cavity.

Kartagener's syndrome   An inherited disorder which results in immobilisation of all ciliated cells, including sperm.

Karyotype   The assessment of the number and quality of chromosomes, usually derived by examination of white cells from the blood.

Laparoscopy   Telescope inspection of the pelvic organs.

Lesch-Nyan syndrome   An inherited disorder affecting boys only. It causes severe metabolic disturbances including kidney failure, and physical handicap.

Luteinising Hormone (LH)   The hormone from the pituitary gland which triggers the final stages of maturation of the egg and ovulation.

Long protocol   Prolonged suppression of pituitary function with drugs – normally for two to four weeks – followed by stimulation of ovarian function.

Lupus anticoagulant   One of the antibodies which may be responsible for failure of an embryo to implant properly, and which may well cause miscarriages.

Magnetic resonance imaging (MRI) or nuclear magnetic resonance (NMR)   A method of creating a three-dimensional image of structures inside the body by getting molecules in the cells to resonate in a powerful magnetic field.

Microinjection   The injection of a single sperm into an egg. See **Intracytoplasmic sperm injection (ICSI)**.

Micron   One hundredth of a millimetre.

Mitochondrium (plural mitochondria)   Tiny bodies present in each cell in the body which carry a part of the DNA, controlling some basic functions, particularly energy usage.

Mosaic embryo   An embryo with varying numbers of chromosomes in each cell.

Mutation   A misprint or change in the structure of a gene – often causing disease.

Myomectomy   Operation to remove a fibroid.

Ovarian hyperstimulation syndrome (OHSS)   see **Hyperstimulation**.

Parthenogenesis   The formation of an embryo – or embryonic-like structure – from an egg which has not been fertilised by a sperm.

Pentoxyfylline   A drug which, when mixed with sperm, sometimes increases their motility.

Percoll   A viscous fluid which acts as a kind of filter and is used to sort cells.

Percutaneous epididymal sperm aspiration (PESA)   Aspiration of sperm through the skin of the scrotum from the epididymis (q.v.) in the testicle.

Pituitary gland   The master gland at the base of the brain which controls many other glands in the body.

Polar body   The small piece of material discarded from a maturing egg which contains one set of unpaired chromosomes.

Polycystic ovary syndrome   A common cause of failure to ovulate. It may also be associated with poor quality eggs when ovulation does occur.

Polygenic   A characteristic or disease caused by a number of different genes working together.

Polymerase chain reaction (PCR)   A diagnostic method for detecting a piece of DNA.

Polyp   A fleshy outgrowth of tissue, commonly in the uterine cavity

Preimplantation embryo   An embryo before implantation in its mother's uterus – essentially the first week or so of embryonic life.

Preimplantation diagnosis   The diagnosis of genetic or other defects in an embryo before implantation.

Progesterone   The female hormone produced by the ovary after ovulation and which primes the uterus to allow implantation of the embryo.

Prostate gland   The gland at the base of the urethra which produces secretions which nourish sperm and which form the seminal fluid.

Recessive genetic defects   A disorder caused when both parents have a similar misprint in a particular gene. Any child born from such parents will have a 1:4 chance of being affected by the disorder.

Recombinant   Genetically engineered (usually refers to a drug).

Releasing hormones (usually LHRH) The hormones which stimulate the pituitary gland to produce (release) gonadotrophins – when used therapeutically the releasing hormone for LH – hence LHRH – may be given.

Salpingolysis Surgical freeing of the fallopian tube.

Salpingostomy Opening the blocked ovarian end of the fallopian tube.

Serum The fluid constituent of the blood from which all cells have been removed.

Sex-linked disorder A genetic disorder which affects a particular gene on the X chromosome. Boys born from a mother carrying an abnormal gene on an X chromosome have a 1:2 chance of being affected by the disease.

Short protocol Brief suppression of pituitary function with drugs – normally for two to seven days – followed by stimulation of ovarian function.

Spermatid Immature precursor of a sperm.

Spermatogenesis The first and main stage of manufacture or production of sperm in the testes.

Synechiae Adhesions sticking tissues together – usually refers to adhesions sticking the internal walls of the uterus together.

Sub-zonal sperm injection (SUZI) Injection of sperm under the outer zona of the end, but not into the cytoplasm.

Tay-Sachs syndrome An inherited recessive disorder. Babies affected by it have severe neurological problems.

Thermography Detection of temperature of the tissues. The testes, when 'overheated' by enlarged veins, may show up as warmer than normal.

Transgenic An animal which has had its genetic structure changed. It passes this new structure on to its offspring.

Thalassaemia An inherited blood disorder causing very severe anaemia, most common in South-East Asia and Mediterranean countries.

Translocation When part of two chromosomes from a different pair get stuck to each other.

Trisomy Three copies of a chromosome instead of the usual pair.

Tuboscopy Examination of the fallopian tube by inserting a fine telescope through its outer (ovarian) end.

Ultrasound   The use of sonar – high frequency sound – to image structures inside the body.

Utriculoplasty   Operation to correct deformity of the uterus.

Vas deferens   The muscular tube which conducts sperm from the epididymis to the urethra, and thence outside the body.

Varicocoele   Enlarged complex of veins, for example around the testes.

Warnock Commission   A government commission set up in 1982 to inquire into issues related to IVF, donor insemination and other aspects of human reproductive treatment. It was chaired by Mary Warnock, the distinguished academic philosopher, now Baroness Warnock.

X chromosome   The sex chromosome of which normal females have a pair – one inherited from the father, one from the mother.

Y chromosome   The sex chromosome which carries the male-determining genes and which is inherited paternally.

Zona pellucida   The gycoprotein 'shell' or coat that surrounds and protects the unfertilised egg, and subsequently the embryo during the first five days after fertilisation.

Zygote   A zygote is a fertilised egg; this term is to some extent interchangeable with the term 'early embryo'.

Zygote intrafallopian transfer   Similar to GIFT (q.v.) except that a zygote is placed in the tube rather than an unfertilised egg.

List of abbreviations

AI   artificial insemination
AID   artificial insemination by donor
AIH   artificial insemination by husband
D & C   dilation and curettage
DI   donor insemination
DMSO   dimethylsulphoxide
FISH   fluorescent *in situ* hybridisation
FSH   Follicle Stimulating Hormone
GIFT   Gamete Intrafallopian Transfer
HRT   hormone replacement therapy
HCG   human chorionic gonadotrophin
HFEA   Human Fertilisation and Embryology Authority
HGAC   Human Genetics Advisory Commission
HMG   human menopausal gonadotrophin
HPRT   hypoxanthine phosphoribosyl transferase
HSG   hysterosalpingogram
ICSI   intracytoplasmic sperm injection
IGF   insulin-like growth factor
ILA   Interim Licensing Authority
IUI   inter-uterine insemination
IVF   *in vitro* fertilisation
LH   luteinising hormone
LHRH   LH-releasing hormone
MRI   magnetic resonance imaging
OHSS   ovarian hyperstimulation syndrome
PCR   polymerase chain reaction
PDG   pre-implanation genetic diagnosis
PESA   percutaneous epididymal sperm aspiration
PZD   partial zona dissection
SUZI   sub-zonal sperm injection
VLA   Voluntary Licensing Authority
ZIFT   zygote intrafallopian transfer

List of UK clinics and the size of their practice

England

Avon

Bath Assisted Conception Clinic
Forbes Fraser Unit,
Royal United Hospital, Combe Park,
Bath BA1 3NG
Telephone 01225 825560

IVF 273 cycles
DI 47 cycles

Southmead General Hospital,
Dept of Infertility
Westbury-On-Trym,
Bristol BS10 5N13
Telephone 0117 959 5102 x 5102

DI cycles 230
IVF Cycles 67

Tower House
22a Somerset Street, Kingsdown,
Bristol BS2 8LZ
Telephone 0117 924 7152

DI Cycles 112

University of Bristol, Centre for
Reproductive Medicine
4 Priory Road, Clifton,
Bristol BS8 ITY
Telephone 0117 902 1100

IVF cycles 730

University of Bristol Division of
Obstetrics and Gynaecology
St Michael's Hospital,
Southwell Street, Bristol BS2 8EG
Telephone 0117 928 5293

New unit

University of Bristol IVF Service
The BUPA Hospital, Redland Hill,
Durdham Down, Bristol BS6 6UT
Telephone 0117 973 2562 x4066

IVF cycles 836

Berkshire

Berkshire Fertility Centre
Belmore Park Surgery,
59a Hemdean, Caversham,
Reading RG4 7SS
Telephone 0118 948 2004

DI Cycles 50

Dunedin Fertility Centre
BUPA Dunedin Hospital,
16 Bath Road, Reading,
Berkshire RG1 6N13
Telephone 0118 958 7676

DI cycles 16

Buckinghamshire

BMI Chiltern Hospital
London Road, Great Missenden,
Buckinghamshire HP16 OEN
Telephone 01494 892 276

IVF cycles 145
DI cycles 23

Cambridgeshire

Bourn Hall Clinic
Bourn, Cambridge C133 7TR
Telephone 01954 719111

IVF cycles 1188
DI cycles 97

The Rosie Maternity Hospital
University Department of Obstetrics
and Gynaecology, Box 223,
Robinson Way,
Cambridge C132 2SW
Telephone 01223 336880

DI Cycles 142

Cleveland

Cleveland Fertility Centre
Spring House, Great Broughton,
Stokesley, Cleveland TS9 71-1X
Telephone 01642 778239

DI Cycles 144

Hartlepool General Hospital
The Cameron Unit, Hartlepool &
East Durham NHS Trust,
General Hospital, Holdforth Road,
Hartlepool TS24 9SH
Telephone 01429 266654

IVF Cycles 135
DI cycles 23

South Cleveland Hospital
Marton Road, Middlesbrough,
Cleveland TS4 313W
Telephone 01642 854856

IVF Cycles 161
DI Cycles 44

Derbyshire

Derby City General Hospital
Fertility Unit, Department of
Gynaecology, Uttoxeter Road,
Derby DE22 3NE
Telephone 01332 625643

DI Cycles 40

Devon

Exeter Fertility Clinic
Royal Devon and Exeter Hospital,
Gladstone Road, Exeter EX1 2ED
Telephone 0139 240 5320

IVF Cycles 58
DI Cycles 294

**Southwest Centre for Reproductive
Medicine**
Ocean Suite Department of
Obstetrics & Gynecology,
Level 06, Derriford Hospital,
Plymouth PL6 8DH
Telephone 01752 763683

New clinic began treatment 10.08.98

Dorset

The Winterbourne Hospital
Herringston Road, Dorchester,
Dorset DT1 2DR
Telephone 01305 263252

DI Cycles 74

Durham

Bishop Auckland General Hospital
Fertility Centre,
Cockton Hill Road,
Bishop Auckland,
County Durham DL14 6AD
Telephone 01388 454034

New clinic with less than 50 DI
treatment cycles. Began treatment
03.03.97

East Sussex

The Esperance Hospital
Hartington Place, Eastbourne,
East Sussex BN21 313G
Telephone 01323 411188

IVF Cycles 282
DI Cycles 275

Essex

Brentwood Fertility Centre
The Essex Nuffield Hospital,
Shenfield Road,
Brentwood, Essex CM15 8EH
Telephone 01277 263263 x403

New DI clinic began treatment
08.06.98

BUPA Roding Hospital Fertility Unit
Roding Lane South, Redbridge,
Ilford, Essex IG4 51DZ
Telephone 0181 551 7107

IVF Cycles 255
DI Cycles 65

Holly House Hospital
Buckhurst Hill, Essex IG9 5HX
Telephone 0181 505 3311

IVF Cycles 333
DI Cycles 45

**North East London Fertility
Services**
Doctor's House, 40 Cameron Road,
Seven Kings, Ilford IG3
Telephone 0181 597 7414

DI Cycles 34

Hampshire

**BUPA Chalybeate/Wessex Fertility
Services**
Chalybeate Close, Tremona Road,
Southampton, Hampshire S016 6UY
Telephone 01703 775544

IVF Cycles 702
DI Cycles 596

The Hampshire Clinic
Assisted Conception Unit,
Basing Road, Old Basing,
Basingstoke, Hampshire RD24 7AL
Telephone 01256 364422

IVF Cycles 68

North Hampshire Fertility Centre
North Hampshire Hospital,
Aldermaston Road,
Basingstoke, Hants RG24 9AN
Telephone 01256 313324

IVF Cycles 23
DI Cycles 118

Herts

Watford General Hospital
Vicarage Road, Watford,
Herts WD1 8HB
Telephone 01923 244366

DI Cycles 123

Humberside

The Hull IVF Clinic
The Princess Royal Hospital,
Saltshouse Road,
Hull HU8 9HE
Telephone 01482 676541

IVF Cycles 286
DI Cycles 135

Kent

BMI The Chaucer Hospital
The Brabourne Suite,
Nackington Road,
Canterbury,
Kent CT4 7AR
Telephone 01227 825100

IVF Cycles 105
DI Cycles 24

BMI Chelsfield Park Hospital
Bucks Cross Road,
Chelsfield, Orpington,
Kent BR6 7RG
Telephone 01689 877855

IVF Cycles 368
DI Cycles 21

Maidstone Hospital
Hermitage Lane, Maidstone,
Kent ME16 9QQ
Telephone 01622 729000

DI Cycles 38

Queen Mary's Hospital
Frognal Avenue, Sidcup,
Kent DA14 6LT
Telephone 0181 302 2678

DI Cycles 3

Leicestershire

Leicester Royal Infirmary
ACU, Ground Floor,
Women's Hospital,
Kensington Building,
Leicester Royal Infirmary,
Leicester LE1 5WW
Telephone 0116 258 5922

IVF Cycles 160
DI Cycles 104

Middle England Fertility Centre
BUPA Hospital Leicester,
Gartree Road, Oadby,
Leicester LE2 2FIF
Telephone 0116 265 3023

IVF Cycles 61
DI Cycles 58

London

Assisted Reproduction and Gynaecology Centre
13 Upper Wimpole Street,
London, W1M 7TD
Telephone 0171 486 1230

IVF Cycles 217
DI Cycles 3

The Bridge Centre
1 St Thomas Street, London SE1 9RY
Telephone 0171 403 3363

IVF Cycles 852
DI Cycles 395

Chelsea and Westminster Hospital
369 Fulham Road, London SW10 9NH
Telephone 0181 746 8585

IVF Cycles 388
DI Cycles 21

The Churchill Clinic
80 Lambeth Road, London SE1 7PW
Telephone 0171 928 5633

IVF Cycles 477
DI Cycles 7

Cromwell Hospital
Cromwell Road, London SW5 OTU
Telephone 0171 460 5713

IVF Cycles 410
DI Cycles 64

The Diana, Princess of Wales Centre for Reproductive Medicine
3rd Floor, Laneborough Wing,
St George's Hospital Medical School,
Cranmer Terrace, Tooting,
London SW1 7 ORE
Telephone 0181 725 3308

New clinic

Guy's and St Thomas' Hospital Trust
7th Floor, North Wing,
St Thomas' Hospital,
Lambeth Palace Road,
London SE1 7EH
Telephone 0171 633 0152

IVF Cycles 651
DI Cycles 66

Hammersmith Hospital
Du Cane Road, London W12 0NN
Telephone 0181 383 3184

IVF Cycles 1180
DI Cycles 11

Homerton Hospital
Homerton Row E9 6SR
Telephone 0181 510 7660/7638

IVF Cycles 150
DI Cycles 27

Dr Louis Hughes
99 Harley Street, London W1N 1DF
Telephone 0171 935 9004

DI Cycles 334

Kings College Hospital
Denmark Hill, London SE5 9RS
Telephone 0171 346 3158

IVF Cycles 930
DI Cycles 136

The Lister Hospital Assisted Conception Unit
Fertility and Endocrine Centre,
The Lister Hospital,
Chelsea Bridge Road,
London SW1W 8RH
Telephone 0171 730 3417

IVF Cycles 1758
DI Cycles 49

London Female and Male Fertility Centre
Highgate Private Hospital,
17–19 View Road, London N6 4W
Telephone 0181 347 5081

IVF Cycles 65
DI Cycles 2

London Fertility Centre
Cozens House, 112a Harley Street,
London W1N 1AF
Telephone 0171 224 0707

IVF Cycles 798
DI Cycles 96

London Women's Clinic
113 & 115 Harley Street,
London, W1N 1DG
Telephone 0171 487 5050

IVF Cycles 507
DI Cycles 221

Multicare International
16th Floor,
1 Harbour Exchange,
Exchange Square, London E14 9GE
Telephone 0171 512 2440

New clinic

Newham General Hospital Assisted Conception Unit
Newham General Hospital,
13 Glen Road, Plaistow,
London E13 8RU
Telephone 0171 363 8069

IVF Cycles 20

The Portland Hospital
214 Great Portland Street,
London W1N 61H
Telephone 0171 390 8262

IVF Cycles 198
DI Cycles 28

St Bartholomews Hospital
West Smithfield, London EC1A 7BE
Telephone 0171 601 7176

IVF Cycles 562
DI Cycles 45

Seymour Clinic, St Mary's Hospital
Ground Floor, Cambridge Wing,
St Mary's Hospital, Praed Street,
London W2 1 PG
Telephone 0171 724 2306

DI Cycles 87

University College Hospital
Private Patients' Wing,
25 Grafton Way, London WC1E 6DB
Telephone 0171 380 9955

IVF Cycles 341
DI Cycles 85

University College London Hospitals Reproductive Medicine Unit,
University College Hospital,
Huntley St, London WC1E 6AU
Telephone 0171 380 9435

New clinic

West Middlesex University Hospital
Twickenham Road,
Isleworth TW7 6AF
Telephone 0181 565 5117

DI Cycles 66

Greater Manchester

Manchester Fertility Services
Manchester BUPA Hospital,
Russell House, Russell Road,
Whalley Range M16 8AJ
Telephone 0161 862 9567

IVF Cycles 706
DI Cycles 420

South Manchester

Billinge Hospital
Upholland Road, Billinge,
Wigan WN5 7ET
Telephone 01695 626 485

DI Cycles 38

St Mary's Hospital Regional IVF Unit
St Mary's Hospital,
Whitworth Park,
Manchester M13 OJH
Telephone 0161 276 6340

IVF Cycles 993
DI Cycles 381

Salford Royal IVF and Fertility Centre
Hope Hospital, Stott Lane,
Salford M6 8HD
Telephone 0161 787 4699

IVF Cycles 205

South Manchester NHS Trust
Withington Hospital,
Nell Lane,
West Didsbury,
Manchester M20 2LR
Telephone 0161 291 4231

IVF Cycles 96
DI Cycles 115

Merseyside

Liverpool Women's Hospital
Crown Street, Liverpool L8 7SS
Telephone 0151 702 4121

IVF Cycles 829
DI Cycles 317

University Hospital Aintree Assisted Conception Unit
Ward 1, Fazakerley Hospital,
Lower Lane,
Liverpool L9 7AL
Telephone 0151 529 3800

IVF Cycles 262
DI Cycles 159

Wirral Fertility Centre
Pine Ridge, Holmwood Drive,
Wirral L61 1AU
Telephone 0151 648 2364

IVF Cycles 99
DI Cycles 57

Norfolk

BUPA Hospital Norwich
Old Watton Road, Colney,
Norwich NR4 7TD
Telephone 01603 255644

DI Cycles 129

Northamptonshire

Northamptonshire Fertility Service
The Cliftonville Suite,
Three Shires Hospital, The Avenue,
Cliftonville, Northampton NN1 5DR
Telephone 01604 601606

IVF Cycles 503
DI Cycles 79

Nottinghamshire

CARE at the Park Hospital
Sherwood Lodge Drive,
Burntstump Count Park, Arnold,
Nottingham NG5 8RX
Telephone 0115 967 1670

IVF cycles 650
DI cycles 49

Nottingham City Hospital
Hucknall Road,
Nottingham NG5 1PB
Telephone 0115 969 1169 x47377

DI Cycles 159

NURTURE
Floor B East Block,
Queen's Medical Centre,
Nottingham NG7 2UH
Telephone 0115 970 9490

IVF Cycles 1245
DI Cycles 24

Queen's Medical Centre Fertility Clinic
University Hospital Queen's
Medical Centre,
Nottingham NG7 2UH
Telephone 0115 970 9238

DI Cycles 153

Oxfordshire

Oxford Fertility Unit
Nuffield Department of Obstetrics &
Gynaecology, Women's Centre,
John Radcliffe Hospital,
Headington,
Oxford OX3 9DU
Telephone 01865 221900

IVF Cycles 887
DI Cycles 76

Shropshire

Shrewsbury and Mid-Wales Fertility Centre
Royal Shrewsbury Hospital,
Mytton Oak Road,
Shrewsbury SY3 8XQ
Telephone 01743 261 202

DI Cycles 48

Surrey

Shirley Oaks Hospital Fertility Treatment Centre
Shirley Oaks Hospital,
Poppy Lane,
Shirley Oaks Village,
Croydon CR9 8AB
Telephone 0181 654 2834

DI Cycles 15

The Woking Nuffield Hospital Assisted Conception Service
Victoria Wing,
The Woking Nuffield Hospital,
Shores Road,
Woking GU21 4BY
Telephone 01483 763 511 x 259

IVF Cycles 163
DI Cycles 27

Tyne & Wear

The Cromwell IVF & Fertility Centre
The Woking Nuffield Hospital,
Kayll Road,
Sunderland SR4 7TP
Telephone 0191 569 9166

DI Cycles 50

Gateshead NHS Trust
Centre for Assisted Reproduction,
Queen Elizabeth Hospital,
Sheriff Hill,
Gateshead,
Tyne & Wear NE9 6SX
Telephone 0191 403 2768

New clinic with less than 50
treatment cycles. Began treatment
17.12.96

Reproductive Medicine Bioscience Centre
International Centre For Life,
Times Square,
Newcastle Upon Tyne NE1 4EP
Telephone 0191 219 4740

IVF Cycles 488
DI Cycles 280

The Washington Hospital Cromwell IVF & Fertility Unit
Picktree Lane, Rickleton,
Washington NE38 WZ
Telephone 0191 417 6463

IVF Cycles 220
DI Cycles 49

West Midlands

Birmingham Women's Hospital Assisted Conception Unit
Birmingham Women's Hospital,
Edgbaston, Birmingham B15 2TG
Telephone 0121 627 2700

IVF Cycles 529
DI Cycles 243

Walsgrave Hospital Centre for Reproductive Medicine
Walsgrave Hospital NHS Trust,
Clifford Bridge Road, Walsgrave,
Coventry CV2 2DX
Telephone 01203 538 874

IVF Cycles 733
DI Cycles 152

Wolverhampton Assisted Conception Unit
Directorate of Obstetrics and
Gynaecology Maternity Unit,
New Cross Hospital,
Wolverhampton WV1 0OW
Telephone 01902 642 880/642 851

New clinic began treatment
20.05.97

Yorkshire

Jessop Hospital for Women
University Research Clinic,
Leavygreave Road,
Sheffield S3 7RE
Telephone 0114 226 8320

DI Cycles 294

Leeds General Infirmary Assisted Conception Unit
Clarendon Wing,
Leeds General Infirmary,
Belmont Grove,
Leeds LS2 9NS
Telephone 0113 292 6136

IVF Cycles 1434
DI Cycles 465

St James's University Hospital
Beckett Street,
Leeds LS9 M
Telephone 0113 206 4612/
206 5387

Sheffield Fertility Centre
24-26 Glen Road,
Sheffield, S7 1RA
Telephone 0114 258 9716

IVF Cycles 634
DI cycles 27

Scotland

Grampian

University of Aberdeen
Department of Obstetrics &
Gynaecology, University of Aberdeen,
Foresterhill, Aberdeen AB9 2W
Telephone 01224 840567

IVF Cycles 643
DI Cycles 292

Lothian

Edinburgh Assisted Conception Unit
Simpson Memorial Maternity Pavilion,
Royal Infirmary of Edinburgh,
Lauriston Place, Edinburgh EH3 9EF
Telephone 0131 536 4260

IVF Cycles 604
DI Cycles 420

Western General Hospital
Crewe Road, Edinburgh EH4 2XU
Telephone 0131 537 1572

DI Cycles 41

Strathclyde

BMI Ross Hall Hospital
221 Crookston Road, Glasgow G52 3NQ
Telephone 0141 303 4855

IVF Cycles 68
DI Cycles 32

**Glasgow Nuffield Hospital Assisted
Conception Unit**
Glasgow Nuffield Hospital,
29 Beaconsfield Road, Glasgow G12 0P1
Telephone 0141 334 9441

IVF Cycles 252
DI Cycles 117

**Glasgow Royal Infirmary Assisted
Conception Unit**
Glasgow Royal Infirmary,
CS Unit, Ground Floor,
Walton Building,
84 Castle Street,
Glasgow G4 0SF
Telephone 0141 211 4428

IVF Cycles 831
DI Cycles 381

Monklands Hospital NHS Trust
Monkscourt Avenue, Airdrie,
Lanarkshire ML6 0JS
Telephone 01236 748 748 x 2087

DI Cycles 269

Tayside

**Ninewells Hospital Assisted
Conception Unit**
Ninewells Hospital and Medical
School,
Dundee DD1 9SY
Telephone 01382 632 111

IVF Cycles 683
DI Cycles 142

Orkney

Balfour Hospital
Scapa Medical Group,
Health Centre,
Kirkwall,
Orkney KW15 1BX
Telephone 01856 885400

No treatments carried out during the
reporting period

Wales

West Glamorgan

Neath General Hospital Sub-Fertility Clinic
Neath General Hospital, Neath,
West Glamorgan SA11 2LQ
Telephone 01639 641161

DI Cycles 24

Singleton Hospital Cromwell IVF and Fertility Centre
Singleton Hospital, Sketty Lane,
Swansea SA2 MA
Telephone 01792 285 954

IVF Cycles 124
DI Cycles 110

South Glamorgan

BUPA Hospital Cardiff
Croescadarn Road,
Pentwyn,
Cardiff CF2 7XL
Telephone 01222 542 720

New clinic

Northern Ireland

Royal Maternity Hospital
Grosvenor Road,
Belfast BT1 2 6BA
Telephone 01232 894633

IVF Cycles 1151
DI Cycles 255

Index